IRRATIONAL MEDICINE

The Antidepressant Crisis And How To Avoid Unnecessary Behavioral Drugs

Jeffrey Wilson

Gracia
Publishing

Irrational Medicine

Gracia Publishing

Copyright © 2004 by Jeffrey Wilson
Printed in the United States of America

All rights reserved,
including the right of reproduction
in whole or in any form.

First Gracia Publishing trade paperback edition 2004

ISBN 0-9763991-1-3

www.irrationalmedicine.com

To contact the author:
jwilson@irrationalmedicine.com

To my mother Ludena Beehler,
and my father Glenn R. Wilson,
who have taught me many lessons.

To my children, John and Jordan,
who continually remind me of
what's important in life.

Irrational Medicine

Contents

1	How I Lost My Golden Ball	7
2	The Wild Man's Cage	17
3	A Dog Goes Down	27
4	Bucketing Out The Pond	38
5	A Vast Abundance Of Needs And Desires	49
6	A Second Wound	63
7	Where Your Wound Is, That's Where Your Genius Is	84
8	Awareness Of An Enemy	101
9	Your Instincts Have Gold In Them	116
10	Can I Have My Golden Ball Back?	141
11	I Look Into My Own Eyes	156
12	A Confrontation With God	173
13	Remove The Demon And You Do Not Need The Exorcist	184
14	The Key	199

Irrational Medicine

The Journey by Mary Oliver

One day you finally knew
what you had to do, and began,
though the voices around you
kept shouting
their bad advice--
though the whole house
began to tremble
and you felt the old tug
at your ankles.
"Mend my life!"
each voice cried.
But you didn't stop.
You knew what you had to do,
though the wind pried
with its stiff fingers
at the very foundations,
though their melancholy
was terrible.
It was already late
enough, and a wild night,
and the road full of fallen
branches and stones.
But little by little,
as you left their voices behind,
the stars began to burn
through the sheets of clouds,
and there was a new voice
which you slowly
recognized as your own,
that kept you company
as you strode deeper and deeper
into the world,
determined to do
the only thing you could do--
determined to save
the only life you could save.

Irrational Medicine

Chapter 1

How I Lost My Golden Ball

Where there is fear we lose the way of our spirit.
- Gandhi

December 2002: I am attending a seminar in Indianapolis Indiana. My roommate is a chiropractor from Cincinnati, Ohio by the name of Jack Armstrong. I have known Jack for a while, and I respect him. One evening after returning to the hotel we are sitting in the room talking. Jack says, "Do you mind if I ask you a question?" I say, "No, go right ahead." Jack, "Well I couldn't help but notice all the pill bottles in the bathroom. Do all those belong to you?" I laugh and say, "Yes, they're all mine." Jack, "What are they for?" I respond, "Well they are to treat my depression. The Wellbutrin and Effexor are antidepressants, the Depakote is a mood stabilizer and provides antiseizure protection, the Buspar is a tranquilizer to help with anxiety and the Concerta is a time-released form of Ritalin for adult ADD." Jack says, "I am amazed that you are on so many pills. How do you function with so many drugs in you?" I say, "I have good days and bad days. My quality of life is alright but I am so tired all of the time probably because of the depression." Jack says, "Have you ever thought about getting off the drugs?" I say, "I have tried in the past but each time my depression returns and the doctor says that proves I have a biochemical

Irrational Medicine

imbalance and need the drugs to survive." Jack says, "Man, someday you might want to try to get off the medicine but be careful because after so many years your body has grown accustomed to having the drugs and will rebel when you try to stop." I say, "It would be nice to get off them. Each month I spend $643 for the pills and it costs me another $120 for a doctor visit. But my doctor says that my depression is a disease and that I will need the drugs for the rest of my life."

How It All Started

I am sure that if I were to ask my parents to list the milestones in my life they would not match my version. They would probably say things like my first day at school, attending Boy Scout camp, etc. But my version of reality is a little different.

Mom Goes to the Hospital

October 1965: I am six years old when my mother is hospitalized for a nervous breakdown. Her room at the Wayne Avenue Mental Hospital is large and tiled, not at all cozy like home. I walk over to her bed, and there she is, this frail woman with her head covered by a sheet. She is a beautiful but sad looking woman of 26. She looks out of place in the bed, as if she were dropped there from heaven. The nurses stay at their station down the hall from the room, and I wonder how I can stay all night with her without being caught. "Mommy," I cry when I reach up to kiss her. "When are you coming home?" I feel myself gasping for air as tears stream down my face. I hug my mother, and she hugs me back weakly, and she says "Hi sweetheart." She doesn't say much more

Irrational Medicine

before we have to leave.

That evening on the way home my brother Garry and I are playing in the backseat of Dad's Chevy Impala jumping up and down like normal four and six year olds. He turns around and yells, "Sit down and shut up. It's your fault your mother's in the hospital." I sit down in the seat and shut up.

The idea that I am powerful enough to put my own mother in the hospital scares me. I decide that I must be a bad person for what I have done to my mother.

The Red Tractor

The day after visiting my mother in the hospital my dad has to return to work. He takes me to the 10 cent store where I pick out the most beautiful red farm tractor. It glistens in the light and has solid rubber tires and a steering wheel that actually works. It is beautiful.

He then takes me to my cousin's house, carries me to a sandbox in the back yard, and sits my new red tractor down beside me. I sit in that sandbox while my Dad walks away from me. Not knowing why I am there, when he might return, or what is going to happen next. But yet I sit in that box and do not even try to get up and go after my Dad. I am doing what I was told. I keep thinking he is leaving me; he doesn't love me anymore because of what I did to my mother.

I am too young to understand that my dad has a lot to worry about right now with his wife in the hospital and two young boys to take care of.

Mom Comes Home

When Mom comes home from the hospital she

Irrational Medicine

is emotionally distant and spends most of her time on the couch. I know all too well that something scary is going on with her, and I feel that I should be able to do something about it. I adapt by becoming tough and independent. Dad spends most of his time working in the basement on projects.

Feeling an exaggerated sense of my own importance I assume everyone is responding to what I do and watching how I behave. I begin to feel responsible for how everything around me turns out – the happiness and suffering of my parents, my grandparents, my friends, and my brother. I learn to judge myself mercilessly and hold myself to a much higher standard than the rest of humanity. Others are allowed to fail, to falter, to seek help; I on the other hand am required to do it all perfectly by myself, without a mistake, without the aid of anyone else. If I think that my true feelings could be disruptive, I learn to conceal them; if someone seems angry or displeased with me, I instantly disown myself and pretend to be whatever they want me to be.

Fear becomes a primary motivator for much of my behavior. It becomes my most familiar and reliable feeling.

Building Bicycle Wheels

My Dad has a knack for mechanical repair and uses that skill to make extra money by repairing bicycles for a major department store. Dad also contracts with his employer to provide them with fully assembled bicycle wheels. He brings home the individual components then the family sits in the basement and assembles the wheels: each of us having a specific task to do. When I first start working I am five years old and make twenty-five cents a night

Irrational Medicine

for placing spokes in the hubs. As I get older I learn to place the first round of spokes in the rim, then the second and third and eventually the entire wheel. As I take on more responsibility my pay increases.

While I am in the basement building bicycle wheels I miss playing with my friends. But it instills in me a strong work ethic, which would pay off later in life and it is a way to spend time with my family.

Hit by a Baseball

July 1968: My cousin Mike and I are throwing a baseball back and forth in my Aunt Ruby's basement when I get hit right between the eyes. The next thing I remember is waking up in the hospital. Luckily it is the same hospital where my Aunt Lucille works. She often stops by to check up on me and to see how I am doing.

I get bored and pull the patches off of my eyes, get out of bed, and make my way toward the fluorescent lights in the hallway. As I approach the doorway, I hear faint voices and see blurry images down the hallway. I walk toward the voices hoping one of them is my aunt. Then a nurse finds me and chastises me for walking the halls.

She picks me up and takes me back to my bed. After I do this several more times the nurses decide to put me in a crib and tie a net over the top to restrain me. But I continue to peel my eye patches back far enough so I can make out where the net is tied and escape.

Despite the setbacks of being caught for some reason I keep trying; I keep fighting for my freedom. This would later prove to be a valuable quality.

Father's Day Present

Irrational Medicine

One year I save my money from building bicycle wheels for several weeks. Mom takes me to Elder Beerman, a local department store, where I buy my father the prettiest leather belt with his first initial G on it for a Father's Day present. A few days after I give him the belt he uses it to whip me. That spanking is especially painful because my own gift has been used to inflict the punishment.

Dad Gives My Dog Away

One day I come home from school and my dog Pete isn't in the back yard waiting on me. Earlier in the week I had been playing around with him while he was eating and Pete snapped at me. He didn't bite me, but it was serious enough that my dad decided that the dog must go.

Dad said that he gave Pete away to a farmer. I never got to say goodbye to Pete; he was my best friend. I am so sad because it's my fault that Pete is gone. I have once again hurt something that I love. What kind of person must I be?

A Southern Baptist For Life

I am brought up in the straitlaced world of the Southern Baptist religion. We go as a family to church every time the doors are open. The sense of God instilled in me by the Southern Baptist faith contains a deep sense of fear, shame, and lack of being good enough. I am taught to be thoughtful of others, circumspect, and restrained in my actions. I learn that it is wrong to desire materialism and that I should be happy with what I have. I am criticized by my parents for wanting too much; whenever I talk

Irrational Medicine

about my dreams I am told – "Don't get too big for your britches." In other words just take what God gives you and be thankful for it.

    I learn that I entered this world with a legacy of evil, and so I must strive and suffer in this world to be redeemed from the iniquity I inherited just by being born. I am routinely exposed to evangelists spouting arguments for my iniquities, lobbying for my damnability. Rarely do I hear biblical references that refer to my magnificence. The term 'faith' always leaves me uncomfortable to hear or use because in my upbringing it is used as a litmus test for spiritual worthiness.

In General

    When I am small my family members rarely, if ever, speak openly of their tender, human feelings. I cannot recall my parents showing any demonstrable signs of love: no hugs, no saying "I love you," no touching. Whenever I don't meet my dad's expectations, he calls me a "playboy" because I act like a child, and he warns "You will never amount to anything." When I feel sad or afraid, I assume I am alone in feeling these things. Since feelings are kept secret, I feel my wounds set me apart from those I love. Throughout all of this I keep my mouth shut and don't speak up for myself. As a child, I feel oppressed and not allowed to be myself at home. I never get angry at my parents for the way I am treated because that would only provoke another beating. I learn instead to turn that violence against myself, constantly criticizing and verbally beating myself up. I treat myself the way my father treats me; judging myself and my feelings as defective and unacceptable.

Irrational Medicine

When the judgments are in full force, I can hardly breathe, choked by the incessant criticism and fear.

The Teenage Years

As a young adult I continue to learn powerful lessons about the kinds of deep pain that can tear at the heart and body. After my last year of grade school my parents sell the house and move to the suburbs. I leave the only friends I know and go to a school full of cliques and middle class snobs. High school is a miserable time.

My dad tries desperately to control my brother and me as we get older and bigger than him. He records our phone calls to see what we are up to. He even tells what few friends I have been able to make to stay away from me because they are a bad influence.

My brother and I discover Dad is having an affair. One evening we are all fighting and my brother jumps in front of the room and says to Mom: "I can't take it anymore. Dad is having an affair." My parents separate and go through a very nasty divorce.

I react to the divorce by feeling emotionally numb. When a friend asks, I respond as if I have no feelings one way or the other. But the toughest part is coming home to an empty house because Dad has moved out and Mom works all the time to try to make ends meet.

A Song on The Radio

October 1980: My brother Garry and I are driving to the Salem Mall to run some errands. The song "Second Hand Rose" by Joe Walsh is playing on the radio. Garry looks at me and says, "I want that

Irrational Medicine

song played at my funeral." I say, "OK" thinking that it will be many years before I would ever have to deal with that issue.

November 1980: My brother Garry, at the age of 18, has an aneurysm burst in his brain while shoveling snow. My father gives him mouth to mouth resuscitation until the paramedics arrive.

Despite doctors' assertions that he will be a vegetable if he survives, I know better. Every time we are allowed to go back and see him I ask him questions, and he responds by squeezing my hand. To me, Mom, and Dad, my brother seems coherent and rational especially considering all of the tubes connected to his head and the respirator he is hooked to.

We have ongoing conflicts with the doctors because they are basically waiting for him to die. I am convinced that they aren't trying hard enough to save him. But I don't know the questions to ask or the buttons to push to get a better response from the doctors. I spend eleven days in a stark waiting room with my parents and their new partners waiting for my brother to get better. There is so much anger between my parents that it fills the room and stifles the air. I feel so alone and helpless while my brother lies in the intensive care unit fighting for his life.

November 29, 1980: It is my grandfather's birthday, and the doctors come out and tell us that my brother is dead.

Afterwards his death doesn't seem real to me. I go through all of the motions in a state of complete shock – my parents and I go to the funeral home and pick out a brown colored coffin that matches my brother's brown Chevrolet Camaro, I purchase a spray of yellow roses for his casket and write his eulogy. I go to the record store and find the song "Second Hand

Irrational Medicine

Rose" to be played at the funeral.

After the funeral I spend the rest of my time alone and bit by bit, begin to understand that the future I have assumed, and the love and support I have come to depend upon, is gone. And there are many, many regrets; for lost opportunities, and a deepening realization that there is absolutely nothing that can be done to change that. The shock of Garry's death gradually disappears over time, but missing him never does.

The accumulated pain and uncertainty from Garry's death, as well as from my parents divorce lowers and narrows my expectations of life. My family, as I have known it, is gone. I stop going to church and start hating God.

Chapter 2
The Wild-Man's Cage

The whole history of science has been the gradual realization that events do not happen in an arbitrary manner, but that they reflect a certain underlying order, which may or may not be divinely inspired.
- Stephen W. Hawking

December 1980: I am grieving the loss of my brother and going through psychospirtual overwhelm. I am struggling with questions, such as the meaning of life and love, the existence of God, and the suffering of others in the wider world. I feel physically exhausted, emotionally abandoned, cry all the time, and frequently miss work. I am experiencing despair, a form of living death.

During a visit with my family doctor he says, "How are you doing?" I say, "I am tired all the time, I don't want to do anything but sit around the house and watch television." After some more questions he says, "You're suffering from depression" I say, "Depression, what's that?" Dr. Clark, "That's when the chemicals in your brain get out of balance." I say, "What causes that?" He says, "We don't know, but antidepressants will bring the balance back." I ask, "How do antidepressants work?" He says, "We don't know, it just works." I thought how odd to be treated for an illness that no one understands, with a pill that no one can explain how it works. He prescribes the antidepressant Desyrel.

Irrational Medicine

I return to work and after several days notice quite a change. When the medicine starts to work the ideas and feelings are fast and frequent like shooting stars. Shyness goes away; the right words and gestures are suddenly there. There are interests found in uninteresting people. Feelings of ease, intensity, power, well-being, and euphoria pervade my being.

With the antidepressant medicine I seem to hardly need any sleep at all. I become a lean mean fighting machine. My mind is always going a mile a minute and I love the feeling of being "charged up." The medicine makes me very bright, energetic. At times I am like a Labrador puppy trampling on people's feelings without realizing and barging into situations at work without thinking first. But my spontaneity and lack of restraint endear me to people and make me an excellent candidate for a supervisory position.

The medicine makes me impatient with life and restless for more. But always, there is a lingering discomfort. I have a terrible temper, and when it erupts it frightens me and anyone near its epicenter. It is the only crack in the otherwise vacuum-sealed casing of my behavior. After each violent outburst, I have to try and reconcile my notion of myself as a reasonably quiet-spoken and highly disciplined person, with an enraged, utterly insane, and abusive man who lost access to all control or reason.

When the medicine is working I am restless, fiery, aggressive, volatile, energetic, risk taking, grandiose, and impatient with the status quo. Of course this serves me well in Corporate America. I so fear losing the positive impacts of the medicine that I religiously take it as prescribed.

At my job I quickly learn that if I work hard and play by the rules, I will be treated well, and I can

Irrational Medicine

pretty much ignore the part of me deeper inside that feels lonely and afraid. I am good at being responsible, a good soldier, honest and industrious. I have high standards, and I am excellent at working autonomously. I work harder for the approval of my superiors than for my own interests. Accompanying these traits are the bad habits of disorganization, procrastination, and perfectionism. I also develop a terrible fear of failure that comes from feeling that I am loved not for myself, but for what I can do. Add to that the difficulty I have relaxing and enjoying myself, and it is a pretty grim picture.

The effort I put in at work is a tremendous one because to me the stakes are high, and my total energy is mobilized and committed to being successful. My worthiness is attained through achievement. Energy that should be available for pleasure and creativity is bound into a way of life that is unfulfilling. I get caught up in a drive for success and fame based on the illusion that it would increase my self-esteem and gain for me the acceptance and approval I seem to need.

As a child I learned to figure everything out myself. I felt it was my job to do everything right, to never ask for help, and to make sure everyone was taken care of. In the process, I learned to feel extremely important – so important that I could not allow anyone to share my burden. As a child I learned to move faster, to hide myself from intimate contact to make myself a moving target, harder to hit. I took refuge in speed, productivity and busyness; camouflaged by relentless activity. I never lingered in one place long enough to be caught. As an adult I stay busy with some task, diversion, or drama, immersing myself in planning, thinking, arranging – anything that will muffle the tender voices, fears and sorrows

Irrational Medicine

that occupy my heart. I also use speed and productivity in my campaign to justify my worth. I learn to work very hard to earn my place, to be allowed to belong somewhere, frantically continuing to accomplish more and more, seeking elusive approval from all the surrogate parents that populate my busy life. Fearing I have not yet accomplished enough, I push harder and faster, taking on additional projects and responsibilities in a desperate drive toward acceptability.

I also try to capture a lasting sense of love and acceptance with my bosses. I put on all kinds of shows for them: I achieve great things, win awards, and pull off amazing projects to get their loving approval. But I never get satisfaction, because these bosses are not my father, nor are they the right men to help me find self-love. I am overly dependent on positive feedback from others and a relentless quest for accomplishment in order to feel good about myself. Because there is really little I can do to influence the behavior of others or to change events, my self esteem is always in danger. Everything I do is with strong determination. Trying so hard leaves me with little pleasure in my life and no joy.

But it all pays off in the material world, because over a seven year period I am promoted five times.

An Official Diagnosis

January 1984: At times it seems as if the medicine is not working, and I go through periods of working too hard but not getting anywhere, often with a frantic, driven, compulsive flavor to my methods. I do not seem to make as much progress as my activity level warrants. But I am afraid to stop, to back off,

Irrational Medicine

take my bearings, and see if I am still headed in the right direction. I wait and wait for the return of the high moods and awesome enthusiasms, but, except for rare appearances, they have given away to anger, despair, and emotional withdrawal. At times I am immobilized by depression, unable to get out of bed, and profoundly pessimistic about every aspect of my life and future. There is a particular kind of pain, elation, loneliness, and terror involved in this kind of madness. When the medicine doesn't work the depression comes back to the surface and I become passive, sensitive, hopeless, helpless, stricken, dependent, confused, rather tiresome, and with limited aspirations.

My family doctor refers me to a psychiatrist who specializes in pharmacology. The psychiatrist tells me that I have a genetic and biological disorder, major depression. To prove it he pulls out a copy of the Diagnostic and Statistic Manual (DSM), the primary tool and bible of psychiatric diagnosis, and reads me a list of symptoms: "The formal criteria for a diagnosis of major depression include a depressed mood or a loss of interest or pleasure in ordinary activities for at least two weeks, accompanied by at least four of the following symptoms:

1. Sad, depressed, or "empty" mood.
2. Loss of interest or pleasure in ordinary activities.
3. Significant weight loss when not dieting, or weight gain, or change in appetite.
4. Sleep disturbances (insomnia, early-morning waking, oversleeping).
5. Activity level slows down or increases.
6. Decreased energy, fatigue.
7. Feelings of pessimism, guilt, worthlessness, helplessness, hopelessness.

Irrational Medicine

    8. Diminished ability to think, concentrate, or make decisions.
    9. Thoughts of death or suicide, suicide attempts. The symptoms must not be due to the direct effects of medications, drugs, or a physical condition, and must not be better accounted for by a grief reaction. The depressed mood is usually self-reported as a feeling of sadness, hopelessness, or discouragement, although it is sometimes denied and may be elicited by a professional interview, or inferred from facial expressions or body language. Some people emphasize physical complaints or report irritability more than sadness."

    The DSM is the professional bible of American psychiatrists and psychologists. It is published by the American Psychiatric Association (APA). It is quite simply a catalog of symptoms. If a patient has enough of the symptoms listed in any cluster, he or she can be "diagnosed" straight from the book – without benefit of lab tests, brain scans, a physical exam, or the taking of a careful medical history.

    After thirty minutes the doctor suggests that I start taking Norpramin instead of continuing with the Desyrel. I say, "I don't care what I take as long as I get back to my old self."

    I am actually relieved at the prospect of having my difficulties prescribed away by an expert. My original feelings of helplessness and "being out of control" are now confirmed by an official medical diagnosis from a genuine psychiatrist. Being officially diagnosed implies that the problem is a disorder or even a brain disease inside of me and totally beyond my control. It's inside me, even a part of me, but I can't do anything about it except to take the prescribed medication. I believe that like a brain tumor, my painful feelings cannot be controlled or

Irrational Medicine

modified by personal understanding or efforts. I never dream of questioning whether the diagnosis is legitimate because the pronouncement is made with so much certainty and authority from the DSM.

The antidepressants help me be who I think I can be. They help me act on my abilities, have the courage of my convictions, live up to my own self-image. So it must be true that I have a biochemical imbalance. I am emotionally helpless and have to have that prescription. My locus of control shifts to the doctor and his prescription pad. My emphasis is on obtaining relief from painful emotions, and bad moods regardless of the potential cost.

February 1984: Tina and I have been dating for six years and the relationship comes to the point where we either get married or go our separate ways. Since I have invested so much time with her, I decide to get married.

At the wedding my mom is still so angry with my dad that she insists that he not be included in the reception line. Since my mom is paying for the rehearsal dinner, I give in to her demand. My dad comes to the wedding but he is mad about not being in the receiving line and does not go to the reception; we do not talk for many years after this incident.

At work my outstanding performance and achievements enable me to maintain the illusion of progress and happiness. I have especially severe standards that apply only to me. In other people, I accept without question thoughts and actions that, in myself, I would consider mean or bad when measured against my ideal standard. Others are allowed to be "ordinary," but I can never be. Throughout all of this I always see myself as a failure.

When my wife complains about my excessive spending and my increasingly angry and

Irrational Medicine

unpredictable moods, I go to the doctor and he increases the dosage of my medicine.

May 26, 1987: My first son, John Ryan, is born and I realize for the first time in my life what unconditional love is. I mellow and decide it's time to talk to my father again. I go to my father's house to show him his grandson. It's been three years since we have talked. He invites us into the house and we have a cordial discussion about the past few years. But nothing is ever mentioned about the incident that caused us to stop talking.

At work my need to justify my existence continues to bring financial rewards. In my mind, I have it that more effort, more work, more money, more power, achievement, promotion, position, cars, a bigger house, prestigious vacations will somehow render me worthy of love and of having life.

December 28, 1988: My second son, Jordan Lynn, is born. It's hard to believe that I now have two children. It just seems like yesterday that the first one was born. I begin to wonder if much of my life is being lived in unreality, with most of my energy devoted to the pursuit of unreal goals. I go to my doctor and he increases my antidepressant dosage again.

Another Relapse

September 1989: I suffer another depressive episode. When I complain of being less lively, less energetic, less high-spirited, my coworkers say "Now you're just like the rest of us." But I compare myself with my former self, not with others. When I am my normal self, I am a hard act to follow. I have become addicted to my high moods. Like gamblers who sacrifice everything for the fleeting but ecstatic moments of winning, or cocaine addicts who risk their

Irrational Medicine

families, careers, and lives for brief interludes of high energy and mood, I find myself craving for the medicine to make the depression go away. This time my doctor discontinues Norpramin and begins Wellbutrin.

Before the new medicine begins to work I wonder which of my feelings are real? Which me is really me? The wild, impulse, chaotic, energetic, and successful one? Or the shy, withdrawn, desperate, suicidal, doomed, and tired one? Once the Wellbutrin starts to act I pick up where I left off. I start working at a frightening pace, putting in ridiculously long hours and sleeping next to not at all. When I go home at night it is a place of increasing chaos with two little children to take care of.

At this point in my existence, I cannot imagine leading a normal life without taking antidepressants.

Something Is Not Quite Right

At work I am now high enough in the organization that I am named in the corporate management succession plan. Upon hearing this, I consider myself to be a "success" for the first time in my life because my superiors think enough of me to plan my future.

My compulsion, my preoccupation with my job is a way to avoid my feelings. As long as I am focused on what is happening out there, I do not have to pay attention to what's happening inside. I continue to concentrate on my goals, achievements, things I can do - never thinking about how I feel. How I feel is like a sewer – somewhere I don't want to go.

As I accomplish more and more I begin to take myself and my work very seriously, until over time I feel increasingly tired, unappreciated, overwhelmed,

Irrational Medicine

and isolated. The more I am convinced my work is important, the less I feel able to ask for the support, sustenance, or company of others. I often make the mistake of thinking that the problems of the entire world are on my shoulders, and it's up to me alone to solve them.

October 1992: My doctor decides that Wellbutrin has run its course and I start taking Paxil.

Chapter 3

A Dog Goes Down

When you try to understand everything, you will not understand anything. The best way is to understand yourself, and then you will understand everything.
- Shunryu Suzuki

July 1993: My depression has resurfaced and my doctor decides to take me off of Paxil and start me on Prozac.

By now Tina and I have been married for eight years and my career is going very well. I travel almost every week, and when I am home I spend a lot of time doing projects around the house, such as building a multilevel deck and laying down a wood floor in the foyer. I enjoy holding and playing with my boys. I am only truly happy when I am with them. I am living the American dream with a wife, two kids, a home in the suburbs, 2 cars, vacations, just like it is supposed to be.

However I begin to notice that when I am home Tina no longer talks about her best friend who is having an affair. She usually keeps me up to date on what her friend has been doing and with whom, but that flow of information stops. When I question her about her friend she just says the affair is still going on, but nothing more. I also realize that Tina no longer complains about my work schedule. She is now totally indifferent to my travels across the country.

Irrational Medicine

One day it occurs to me that maybe Tina has decided to try what her best friend is doing. I begin to have a nagging feeling, an intuitive feeling, that something is wrong so I start to secretly record telephone conversations at the house.

Betrayal

December 1993: My telephone recording goes on for several weeks and I barely have time to listen to the tapes in between my travels. But one afternoon I am reviewing a call between Tina and her best friend when she casually asks, "How is it going with Jim?" A simple enough phrase that literally destroys my world. Tina responds: "He is OK, we're seeing each other on Thursday." I turn off the tape recorder and just stare into space. In an instant my entire world comes crashing down around me. My body begins to convulse and shake as the words "He's OK" echoes in my head. At that moment my view of the world and all its problems, pleasures, and distractions change instantly.

A thousand thoughts a second flood my mind. How can my wife do this to me, what will my family and friends think? Then I collapse on the bedroom floor unable to speak. What seems like hours pass before I finally regain my composure.

I am not sure what to do, so I keep this to myself for several weeks while I try to sort out what is happening. I go ahead with our plans to attend a New Year's Eve party at a local hotel with some friends.

December 31, 1993: We check into the Embassy Suites in Blue Ash with our friends Joe and Janet about 7:00 p.m. As the evening wears on I start feeling like a caged animal. I can't look at Tina without feeling anger rage inside of me. Because it is

Irrational Medicine

New Year's Eve we are drinking alcohol, which doesn't help me maintain my composure.

After dinner Tina and I go back to our hotel room to get ready for the dance that will ring in the New Year. While we are sitting in the room I blurt out "How is Jim?" She looks at me as if she has seen a ghost. I say, "I know about your affair, do you want to confess?" After a few minutes she begins to say he is a friend. I can tell by her tone on the tapes as well as her discomfort in the moment that he is much more than a friend. So I play along like I have more information than I do to try to trick her into telling me what is going on. Finally she admits that she is having an affair with him. I don't want to know any of the details, I have heard enough.

January 1994: Over the next several days Tina and I manage to have somewhat civil conversations. Although several times I lose control and kick and punch closet doors and walls. I am so angry at her lack of concern for her family and how she can put at risk everything I have worked so hard for. Eventually Tina agrees to stop seeing Jim, and go to marriage counseling.

With each passing day I slip into a deeper state of depression. At the end of January my doctor increases my dosage of Prozac.

Tina and I start going to a marriage counselor once a week. In addition, we each go to individual therapists by ourselves. Instead of going on a normal vacation to the Smokey Mountains we attend a Marriage Encounter retreat. Later we take a cruise to celebrate our wedding anniversary, and I buy her the diamond eternity ring she has always wanted.

Meanwhile my performance at work starts to slide. I have lost the love of my job and can't stay focused long enough to get anything accomplished. I

Irrational Medicine

try to act concerned but I am too miserable to care. I feel duty bound, but I am so absorbed in my own depression and misery that I almost hate my employees for burdening me with their problems.

One day we experience major problems in the computer network. Usually there is nothing like a genuine crisis to rally me out of a bad mood, to snap me into a "get things done" mode, but I am so far gone at this point that the special surge of necessary energy, the adrenaline rush, is not hitting me at all. I am simply plodding along, forcing myself to care. I hate myself for being so low, and I hate the people around me for needing me to be otherwise.

The doctor increases my dosage of Prozac and warns me that it is at the maxim level he is comfortable with. I wait and wait for the return of good moods and enthusiasm, but except for rare appearances, all I can manage is anger, despair, and bleak emotional withdrawal. At times I am immobilized by depression, unable to get out of bed, and profoundly pessimistic about every aspect of my life and future.

July 1994: My boss and I have a talk about my performance. For the first time since entering the adult work force I am told that my performance is not up to standard. He says that he has seen a dramatic change in my style and attitude at work and is concerned about my future. I am absolutely shocked by this meeting and it sends me even further into depression.

August 1994: My moods are even worse so the doctor stops the Prozac and starts me on Zoloft. The doctor tells me that this drug will start working in a week or two, but he doesn't understand that I don't have a week or two. He obviously doesn't understand that the pain is so bad that I don't want to live like

Irrational Medicine

this anymore.

September 1994: Things have settled down at home and the counseling seems to be helping our marriage so I start to travel out of town again. After a few weeks that nagging feeling returns, so during a trip to New York I have a private detective follow Tina for the day - the results are devastating. He calls me in New York to tell me that Tina met Jim at our neighbors house (she was house sitting while they were on vacation) and spent the afternoon with him there.

I just sit in my hotel room in shock. I have spent ten months in a living hell trying to rebuild my marriage. I have tried everything I know to save my marriage and put my life back together but it just isn't enough. I feel that all the counseling, the trips, the gifts, time, and money were for nothing. I have been betrayed again. Now I am finished. I will not waste another ounce of energy or time or any other resource on trying to save this marriage. Tina has clearly made her decision and I am not going to argue with it.

I change my flight to leave New York a day earlier and I spend the next several hours on the telephone locating an apartment, and a moving company. I also call my mother and some friends of mine and tell them to meet me at the house the next day to help me move out. The next day when Tina comes home from work she discovers that I have left her and taken one half of everything in the house.

Alone Again

October 1994: My depression is really deep now. The doctor adds Lithium and raises my dosage of Zoloft. But I am on a slippery slope and nothing is stopping me. I still keep taking the medicine because I

Irrational Medicine

am told to, but it does not provide any meaningful protection against the terrible agitation and pain within my mind. I keep telling the doctor that the antidepressants are not working quickly enough. And he says, "Give it time." God do I wish that he could know what it's like to be a patient and to feel so desperate.

After several weeks it begins to dawn on me just what has really happened. I have lost my marriage, my family. I am not seeing my two beautiful boys each night and tucking them in bed and kissing them goodnight. I am sleeping alone for the first time in nine years. My life has changed so dramatically. Everything I have worked so hard for is gone. My dreams are shattered. In addition to the mental strain of a dissolving marriage and a failing career, my family doctor tells me I need to have my gall bladder removed.

At work my performance is still bad, but I apply for a new position in strategic planning. Based on my past history and some favors, I get the job. It has the potential to be a great move if I perform well, but I can't muster any enthusiasm and totally neglect my new duties. I feel as if I am dying day by day, emotionally and mentally. I have lost my zest for life and my will to live. I have given up. I am seeing my doctor weekly now and he increases the dosage of the Zoloft and Lithium almost every visit. But nothing helps me, nothing.

January 1995: I have been warned several times but finally my boss has had enough. I am fired from the company I have devoted so much of my life to. It is not a surprise but I am disappointed. Now everything is gone, my wife, my family, my job, everything I have worked so hard for all these years is gone.

Irrational Medicine

After being fired I don't have to be personable for anyone. Now the despair really has a chance to surface. I start feeling this uncontrollable sadness and disconnect from most of the people in my life. I have no energy to deal with them or their problems.

I have counted upon my mind's sharpness, interest, reliability and now, all of a sudden, my mind has turned on me. It no longer finds anything interesting or enjoyable or worthwhile. It is incapable of rational thought and turns time and again to the subject of death: "I am going to die anyway, what difference does anything make? My life's run is only a short and meaningless one. I am totally exhausted and can scarcely pull myself out of bed in the mornings, why live?"

As I sit on the balcony of my apartment overlooking the pond, I think about how suicide could make all these thoughts, all my problems go away. In one fell swoop my problems would be gone. After all without my children with me, or my job, or my beautiful house what is there to live for. I begin to plot out the logistics of putting a gun in my mouth and pulling the trigger.

I am truly at the bottom, unsure of how or even if I want to pick up the pieces of my broken life. When I finally recognize the madness of these thoughts I go see my therapist John Bender. After I explain my desire to commit suicide. He says, "When a person commits suicide, it means he cannot live with himself. He can no longer endure the negative and hostile feelings within and he cannot express these feelings except through some destructive act." I say, "So what." He continues, "If you commit suicide you will be giving your children permission to deal with their problems the same way." That statement hits me very hard. I never considered the impact of my actions on my children. At that moment I decide that suicide will never be a real option for me.

When I leave John's office I drive directly to Good Samaritan Hospital in Cincinnati and check myself in to their mental illness Day Treatment Program.

Going To The Hospital

On my first day in the program a treatment team is assigned to me consisting of a psychiatrist, a clinical psychologist, a nurse, a recreational therapist, an occupational therapist, and a clinical social worker. During the first day I meet with the entire team and they conduct a comprehensive assessment and establish my treatment goals. The program schedule is from 8:00 a.m. to 2:00 p.m. Monday through Friday. I am assigned a locker where I can keep my personal belongings and I am expected to eat lunch with the other participants in the program in the hospital cafeteria. The program consists of a number of group and self-directed activities. There are also reading assignments that I have to do every day.

The therapists use an approach in group called cognitive therapy, which focuses on how we think. It emphasizes replacing self-defeating ideas or concepts with more positive and effective ones. Their goal is to help the patients learn how to heal and protect ourselves during conflict and how to remain independent within loving relationships. During the daily group sessions, I sit in the circle listening to the hopelessness of the other people in the program.

During breaks I walk down the hall and look at the inpatient treatment program that is right next door; often feeling that I am only one breath away from being in there.

Irrational Medicine

Each day we have Work/Task Skills Group or as I call it arts and crafts. It is my favorite time of the day because I don't have to listen to the depressing stories of the other people in the group and can just work by myself. I get to create things with my hands, something I never do at my job because all of that work is mental. During my time in the program I produce a wooden stationary box, which I paint hunter green, a miniature apple crate, and my favorite item, which is a small wooden stool. I assemble the frame consisting of four wooden legs and cross supports. Then I paint the frame hunter green. Once that is complete I weave a thirty foot single piece of rattan through the frame to make the seat top. (To this day this stool is in my office at home to remind me of just how low my life had gone. When I look at it I can instantly recall the despair, the fear, the sheer loneliness that consumed me during this time in my life. The stool serves as a reminder of exactly where I will never go again.)

In the group therapy session the question comes out: "Are you depressed because you have lost your wife's love?" I say, "No, I am depressed because I don't have my children with me or live in the home I worked so hard for. I am depressed because I couldn't conceive that my wife could turn to another man. I am depressed because my dreams are shattered."

After several weeks I still feel completely drained and sleep 10-12 hours a night. For a long time, all I care about is going to sleep and don't really care if I wake up the next day. I don't have even a dim awareness of a potentially better life. I am swimming in a lake of helplessness and hopelessness, paralyzed in my ability to make satisfying or meaningful choices. I fear there are no viable alternatives; no choices that will make any real difference, and that

Irrational Medicine

ultimately I must in some way bear the blame for my fate.

Basically My Last Chance

February 28, 1995: During a session with my therapist he asks me how the Day Treatment Program is going. I say, "I feel like I have made very little progress in the program but sometimes I have the strangest feeling that I don't really want to leave the hospital. The prospect of going back into the real world, with its constant demands that I be responsible, is terrifying."

John says, "That's understandable because when life has driven someone to feel so overwhelmingly helpless it may take time and effort to find the understanding, direction, motivation and courage to climb out of the darkness." I say, "The experience is character building, but I am beginning to tire of all the opportunities to build character at the expense of a normal life. My self-confidence, which has permeated every aspect of my working adult life, is no longer there. The damn antidepressants are not doing their job. I am taking ever increasing dosages of Zoloft and Lithium but they don't make me feel better." John snaps at me, "Do you expect the drugs to make you feel better, to fix your problems?" I say, "Well yes, I have a biochemical imbalance, it's a disease." John says, "You are expecting the drugs to do too much. There are underlying emotional issues that you need to address rather than relying on the medicine to make you functional. With that attitude it's no wonder you're not making progress at the hospital. You have the depressing idea that your life offers no worthwhile alternatives, you need a change in attitude, not a mind altering drug. You have

Irrational Medicine

feelings such as hopelessness and despair that are undermining your life, you need to find encouragement and hope. You don't need to have your feelings artificially blunted or elevated by a drug. You need to find new ways of thinking and feeling about your life, and ultimately, you need a new approach to making choices that are more ethically consistent and fulfilling." He hands me a brochure for a personal growth seminar called Basic, sponsored by Life Success Seminars and says, "You obviously need something drastic to snap you out of this. I strongly urge you to attend one of their Basic seminars."

The next day my psychiatrist finally gives up on the drug combination of Zoloft and Lithium ever working and puts me back on Wellbutrin. Later that day I read the Basic brochure that John gave me. I have been to many business seminars but I never knew there was training for "personal growth." I put the brochure aside but keep coming back to it. There is a strange pull for me to go, like a still small voice urging me on. Finally I decide that since the medicine isn't working, and intensive hospital therapy every day isn't working, what do I have to lose by going to a seminar for four days. I have the attitude that if this Basic seminar doesn't work, my life is over; it's my last chance. So I call Life Success Seminars and register for the March training. Little do I realize that I am about to meet my teacher.

Chapter 4

Bucketing Out The Pond

Darkness cannot drive out darkness; only light can do that. Hate cannot drive out hate; only love can do that. Hate multiplies hate, violence multiplies violence, and toughness multiplies toughness, in a descending spiral of destruction. The chain reaction of evil must be broken, or we shall be plunged into the dark abyss of annihilation.
- Dr. Martin Luther King Jr.

March 1995: I rarely feel comfortable when I encounter people who offer tenderness and love. When I walk into the hotel where the Basic seminar is being held and meet the registration staff all I see is tenderness and love. My first thought is perhaps they are after something, or maybe they are just in denial. I am sure that their kind words conceal some danger or criticism just below the surface. Walking into the main meeting room I really have my guard up as the seminar begins.

The man leading the seminar is Jim Quinn, the founder of the LifeStream organization. He explains that the seminar is experiential, which means we will be up and moving around a lot with a little lecture from time to time. He explains the weekend is filled with exercises designed to teach specific lessons about life. He reviews the ground rules and takes questions from the audience.

I stand up and challenge Jim. I say, "Sometimes I feel entitled to be depressed and angry. I

Irrational Medicine

have suffered a lot of crap in my life, and if anyone deserves to be angry, it's me. I have been depressed for so long that it feels safe and comfortable. Like an old blanket I keep myself warm at night with all my grievances. It's easy, quiet and unchallenging. I can stay home, watch TV, and feel sorry for myself. It is easier than working my way out of it."

Jim says, "When you're green you grow, when you're ripe you rot. The path you're on is not static. Once you start rotting you don't stop. It's a slippery slope down to despair. You may be able to watch a few weeks of TV safely, but any more than that and your self-esteem, ambition, humor, and creative juices dry up. Before long you have trouble leaving the house at all. You'll stop answering the phone. Pretty soon you'll put your head in the oven." I think, wow he really nailed me, as I sit down without admitting that I am already there. I decide to listen to what this man has to say. While I do not fully realize what is going to happen over the next four days, the decision to start listening opens the gates to enormous personal growth.

A Whole New World

During the first evening I learn that I am not broken, that my childhood suffering is not a mortal wound and it does not irrevocably shape my destiny. For the first time I begin to understand that no one hurt me so badly that I cannot heal. I learn that it is all right to accept my feelings and whatever information they contain, that contrary to my usual belief, the shame from childhood had not annihilated my abilities and talents. I may feel empty, numb, and entirely without feelings, but that is not reality. My longing for a better life reveals that something inside

Irrational Medicine

me (that still, small voice), has always remained alive, has always been perfectly aware of what I need, and has been seeking it intensely, for quite a long time.

My challenge is not to try and repair what is damaged but instead to reawaken what is already strong and whole within me, to cultivate the qualities of heart and spirit that are available to me. I leave the Thursday evening session ready to come back Friday, Saturday and Sunday and fight for my life.

The Teaching Continues

Throughout the next three days Jim uses insightful educational techniques to facilitate my understanding of the suffering in my life. I participate in every exercise 100 percent. I am the last to leave the room at breaks and the first to be back in the room when the seminar starts again. I sit in the front row and pay very close attention to everything Jim says and does. I learn many, many lessons.

Jim reviews numerous concepts, such as there are only two ways our lives can improve. The first way is that everyone else changes how they treat us. The second is that we change how we react to other people. Since the chance of getting everyone else to change the way they treat me doesn't seem very possible, I go with number two.

Jim talks about our true nature being more like that of a young child before all the stuff builds up around our hearts. A young child is naturally joyful, loving, peaceful, trusting, energetic, and creative, and we can be too. But over time the world intrudes on us, and we become "normal" – angry, apathetic, insecure, fearful, reactive, and anxious.

In one of the few lecture portions of the weekend Jim spends time describing the four basic

Irrational Medicine

human natures: Physical, Mental, Emotional, and Spiritual. He says, "If any one of these is out of balance we feel it in our lives. Some of our Physical needs are food, water, diet, exercise, rest, and physical activity. Some of our Mental needs are reading, intellectual challenge, and rest. Some of our Emotional needs are hugs, being with people who love us and encourage us, to love and to be loved. Some of our Spiritual needs are play, creativity, prayer, music, art, charity, poetry, the need to love and to be loved. Seeing that we get our basic needs met and keeping them in balance is a vital part of a productive and happy life. Having a balance between these four natures is the key to peace."

One of the key exercises of the weekend for me is dealing with forgiveness. Through this process I forgive my parents for the violence, the abandonment, and the divorce. I see them not as evil, but as people who could not manage to honor and cherish their own children, their own spouse, or their own lives in a loving and gentle way. I forgive their suffering, their confusion, their unskillfulness, their desperation, and their humanity. I also forgive my brother for dying and leaving me alone. I forgive myself for being the only child of three who survived. I am set free from the cycle of suffering when I forgive others and allow them to be who they are, nothing more, nothing less. They were less than the ideal mother or father perhaps, but children of God still, with all their suffering and distress, who need all the grace and mercy available to them. Through forgiveness I am set free to go my own way and follow my own destiny.

In another lecture portion of the training, Jim describes a different view of depression. He explains: "Depressed people have a leak in part of the self that contains a positive, nurturing self-image. Instead of

Irrational Medicine

having a good opinion of themselves – a reservoir of self-esteem – that can be sustained through the difficulties of life, they are overly dependent on love, respect, and approval from significant people in their lives. Sometimes they are not so visibly dependent on others, but on the symbols of love, respect, and approval – financial success, control, power. Therefore a loss or threat to these relationships or symbols can precipitate a depression in people who have been functioning quite well when these relationships were stable, and can make a depression much worse in people who have had depressive symptoms already."

I realize that I must learn to practice self care and provide my own esteem. What this means is a deliberate effort to practice the skills I am learning in the seminar, changing how I am in relationships, assessing my priorities and trying to live in accordance with my values. It also means letting myself feel proud of my accomplishments.

Insights and realizations continue to fly into my head and heart. I learn a wonderful meditation technique to calm and still my mind. I also learn the difference between being responsible for myself and to someone else. Most importantly I learn that not only is it important to love others but to love myself. What a new concept for me, I am allowed to love and care for myself.

I begin to understand that I have not lived with much emotion. Other than when my children were born or someone died, I am very flat emotionally. My head is alienated from my heart; I have been dead from the neck down. It is a relief to me that things I am accustomed to choking off, such as tears, can be recognized and taken seriously. I realize how I have been forced to look for distraction in work, projects at home, or watching TV, when I am moved, upset, or

Irrational Medicine

sad.

Yes, I suffer from depression, but more importantly I am undergoing a psychospiritual crisis, surrounding issues of basic identity and shame with feelings of outrage and overwhelmedness. The meditation helps me with this by calming my mind and letting me feel my heart.

Throughout the four days Jim Quinn gives me love and guidance in a way that I have never experienced. He respects me and sees worth in me that no one else has ever acknowledged. I feel accepted and whole, nurtured and good – feelings that I had given up long ago.

Jim teaches me that it is alright to love myself and other people. His teaching changes my perceptions of the world and opens me up to personal and psychological growth. His words touch a chord inside of me that has long been painfully silent. It is the chord of the awakening of my soul.

I leave the training with an understanding of new principles of living and a new commitment to spiritual and philosophical ideas. On Sunday afternoon, when the seminar is over, I run into the registration people from Thursday night. They literally do not recognize me. I have released so much anger that I have physically changed over the four day period.

I know that my life will never be the same. Reaching out to Jim Quinn became my first step back to human reality. When he responded with love and care, my recovery process began. Without a doubt, Jim Quinn is responsible for saving my life.

My Next Step

I immediately sign up for the next level of

training which is called Inter Personal Intensive (IPI). It is five days long and is held at a retreat center outside of Cincinnati. The next IPI is in three weeks, and nothing can stop me from being there.

For the first part of the week, I am uptight and phony. My ego is threatened because it knows I must give up my old way of being, and that is something the ego does not easily relinquish. During the first two days I risk little, but watch very carefully. I see that when people drop their guard and confess their fears and failings, they are not shamed, but rather supported and held through the experience. What's more, they seem to emerge stronger and with more self respect, not less.

At IPI I get the first idea that my own childhood could have been considered abusive. During a group session, facilitator, Steve Sherwood asks me to describe my childhood, especially how I am disciplined. He says, "Do you think that is abuse?" I say: "No, It was merely a punishment. My parents were doing the best they knew in order to raise me; I can't blame them." Steve says, "You're right, It is not a blame game. But there are basically four types of abuse: physical; sexual; psychological (which includes witnessing spouse abuse); and physical and emotional neglect (not what they do but what they don't do). Psychological abuse can take the form of name calling, humiliation, rejection, putdowns, being degraded, being belittled, being made to feel ashamed of oneself, isolation, and witnessing marital violence. The emotional effects of abuse can cause a person either to experience overwhelming feelings or to have trouble identifying them at all. Feeling-reactions include: anger, sadness, loneliness, hopelessness, fear, anxiety, and depression. Two common reactions to childhood abuse are low self-esteem and distrust of

Irrational Medicine

self and others."

Right away I start to rationalize the hurt, to minimize and deny the abuse by saying: "I was a difficult child to raise. I never used to listen to my parents. It was just normal punishment. They both worked very hard to put food on the table and were stressed out. They would whip me only when I gave them good reason - I asked for it. They were just trying to bring me up right. It taught me the difference between right and wrong, and it made me stronger." Steve says, "There are also behavioral reactions, which are the outward manifestations of feelings and attitudes. These include destructive behaviors, such as violence, addictions, issues relating to sexuality, money, and self care. Anger is one of the most common reactions to having been abused. Ordinarily anger tells us that we are uncomfortable with a situation and motivates us to respond appropriately." I say, "I was never able to express my anger directly to my parents because it only increased the likelihood of getting hit. I was taught that getting angry was inappropriate, disrespectful, just plain wrong."

Steve says, "The anger doesn't go away by itself: it sits and festers. And over time that anger turns into rage and gets harder to ignore. If you feel uncomfortable with your anger, you will purposefully try to avoid situations that make you feel more anger. Gradually your goal becomes not to feel or show anything. This pattern may be so automatic for you that you lose touch with your feelings altogether. You are sick and suffer because your parents were sick and suffered. They were sick and suffered because their parents were, and so on. The problem is a multi-generational illness or chain of unhealthy learned behaviors and that thinking must be broken or those behaviors and unhealthy thinking will continue down

Irrational Medicine

through the generations. They were unable to recognize the abuse as such and passed it on to you in turn, without even a trace of a bad conscience. You must face and understand what happened to you, or you will create a similar unhealthy atmosphere for your children."

At that moment something shifts inside of me and I promise that I will never beat, whip or spank my children ever again. Instead of trying to constantly control my children I will develop empathy for them. I am determined to be a father who is active and involved, happily part of their lives, a father who is his own man and also teacher to his kids. The cycle of abuse stops with me.

As the week progresses I begin to remember with feelings of rage and helplessness, of anger and indignation, how humiliated and deserted I felt when I was spanked by my father. They were feelings that I could never experience overtly but nevertheless carried all these years. I absorbed countless insults, criticisms, and judgments, and these voices found a home in my psyche, and for most of my life they have served as my intimate companions. I begin to understand that as a child it was difficult for me to learn self-esteem when my true self was rejected in such a painful way, that I did not trust that anyone could ever truly love me if my family rejected me, that I have been permanently ashamed, that fears bind energy, and that over time I have successfully constructed strategies to protect myself.

Steve teaches, "It's not life's inevitable tragedies that stifle, overwhelm us, and cause us so much pain. It's the "stuffing" of them that does us in. So let yourself feel what you feel. Learn what your needs are, and get them met in healthy and loving ways. Each one of us is responsible for getting our needs

Irrational Medicine

met. We set ourselves up for major disappointments when we depend too heavily on any one person to meet our needs."

I learn that in a healthy person, feelings constantly change. One can be angry, then loving, sad, then joyful. Each strong feeling creates a new direction that is the person's personal response to their environment. All true emotions have this personal quality. They are direct expression of the life forces within the person - faith can be seen as an aspect of feeling. The more one feels, the stronger is his faith. My chief shortcoming in my personal relationships is a lack of awareness of my own emotions and my blindness to the emotions of others.

As the week progresses and I participate fully in the exercises, something marvelously thrilling happens inside of me. I feel as if a warm and wonderful sun is rising in my chest. The spirit of the seminar appeals to a deeper and more satisfying level of my being than I have experienced since I was a little child. Steve shows me that life is much more satisfying when we are open, honest, accepting, trusting and loving.

IPI turns out to be all that I wanted, expected and needed – and more. At the end of the week my heart flies open with the possibility of the reality of love and happiness and a purpose for life. My relationship with God is rekindled. I step out of the loneliness of isolation and into the warm sun of a life worth living.

The day after IPI ends I go back to Good Samaritan Hospital in Cincinnati and check myself out of the outpatient mental health program. The other patients in the program see me and will not let me leave until I tell them where I have been and what I have done that has changed me so much. I explain

Irrational Medicine

about the Basic and IPI seminars and say, "Basic stopped my downward spiral into depression by showing me a different way to live. It allowed me to crack the shell of indifference that covered my authentic self. IPI allowed me to break through the shell and access parts of me that I had forgotten a long time ago. I can now give up the chronic, never-ending, corrosive state of victim-hood. IPI and Basic encourage self-determination, taking responsibility for the consequences of one's actions, and living by more fulfilling psychospiritual values. My experience at Basic and IPI was worth 10 years of psychotherapy. I got in touch with my feelings, and my inner being. It restored my faith in myself and made me an inner-directed person. Overcoming trauma and moving forward is liberating." I then give each member of my group a brochure and a hug as I say goodbye.

Chapter 5

A Vast Abundance Of Needs And Desires

Everything you see has its roots in the unseen world. The forms may change, yet the essence remains the same. Every wonderful sight will vanish; every sweet word will fade, But do not be disheartened, The source they come from is eternal, growing, Branching out, giving new life and new joy. Why do you weep? The source is within you And this whole world is springing up from it.
- Jelauddin Rumi

Immediately after IPI I begin to experience fantastic changes in my life. I begin to journal and to be turned on by people. I can touch others, physically and emotionally. I speak my truth in all my relationships. My life is evolving at a fantastic pace. New and exciting relationships blossom almost overnight. I meet my IPI buddies socially at least once a week, sometimes more. I just want to live, and to grow and to experience this wonderful feeling of being alive because it is so new to me. As each day passes I continue to integrate the lessons I have learned from Basic and IPI. My mental condition improves and my outlook on life is better. I have never felt so good. It's like the garbage is cleaned out of my system. I am in love with life and life is in love with me.

May 1995: I go back through the Basic seminar but this time as a Team Leader. I find it helpful to repeat the training because I am mentally

Irrational Medicine

in a different place than I was back in March and I hear the lectures and participate in the exercises from a different perspective.

June 1995: Tina and I meet at the county courthouse to finalize our divorce. As we're sitting in the waiting area I am quite comfortable with what is about to happen. I want the divorce to be over with so I can move on with my life. The judge awards us shared parenting. This means the boys live with me one week and their mother the next. This works out great because the weeks I don't have them I see them anyway during their baseball or football games. It is the next best thing to having them all the time. For them the benefit is that each parent is very involved in their lives. I buy them enough clothes and toys so they don't have to carry things back and forth between their mother's apartment and mine. They get two of everything.

July 1995: I repeat IPI as a Team Leader.

August 1995: I feel so good that I tell my psychiatrist that I want to stop taking the antidepressant medicine. He reluctantly agrees to let me taper off my dosages and see what happens. Over the next couple weeks I take less and less of the medicine each day. A few days after stopping completely I become overwhelmed with exhaustion, anxiety and agitation. It is so debilitating that I start the drug again and am immediately relieved. (It never occurs to me that this is really a drug withdrawal reaction.) My doctor misinterprets the response as reemergence of my depression – and says that this is evidence of the effectiveness of the drug and that I must have it to fight off depression. He says: "You will need to be on antidepressants for the rest of your life."

September 1995: I receive a job offer from a major hotel chain headquartered 85 miles away in

Irrational Medicine

Columbus, OH. Moving away is a difficult decision because I will not be close to my children but my money and prospects for employment in Cincinnati are running out. I accept the job but in order to stay connected to my children I make the drive between Columbus and Cincinnati every weekend and frequently during the week to attend their little league baseball or football games. I usually try to leave work a couple hours early each Friday afternoon so I can be in Cincinnati in time to get them off the school bus. Then I drive them back to Columbus for the weekend. Then back to Cincinnati on Sunday evening. Each weekend I put 340 miles on my car.

After relocating to Columbus one of the first things I do is find a new psychiatrist, Dr. Wallen. Because of my dependence on antidepressants I fear not having access to the medicine.

At work I uncover a major technical challenge and launch a 6 month project to revamp the company's infrastructure. It's a huge project costing millions of dollars and has serious ramifications if I fail to pull it off. I love it because this is the type of work I am best at.

November 1995: I go back to Cincinnati and participate in another IPI as a Team Leader. Again I am at a different place in my life and I find the training helpful with my thoughts, feelings and beliefs.

April 1996: I finish my big infrastructure project under budget and two days ahead of schedule. It is so successful that the company issues a press release, I am interviewed by an industry trade magazine and I get a promotion. Finally my career is back on track.

July 1996: I find out that there is an organization in the Columbus area that sponsors a

Irrational Medicine

Basic seminar every few months. I call Susan Estep, the City Director, and volunteer my services to help out any way I can. She gladly accepts my offer for the Basic seminar coming up in a few weeks. I work with Susan for the four days and start a wonderful friendship with her. She is a bright, enthusiastic and cheerful woman. I also meet Ross Quinn, the founder's son because he is leading the Basic. Susan tells me about Ross's training called LeaderShape and how much fun she had going through it. I have been looking for something beyond IPI, something different and challenging. This sounds like it so when I return to work on Monday I convince my boss to send me to the August LeaderShape training.

August 1996: The training is held at Lake Geneva, Wisconsin and is a blend of experiential education and adventure education. During the day we tackle ropes course challenges and at night we study Mother Teresa and Buckminster Fuller. It is a fun and safe environment that encourages personal risk taking. Ross teaches me how to recognize the differences between the fears associated with real risks and perceived risks. There is an unforgettable day of rock climbing at Devil's Lake and it is a profound week of physical, mental, emotional and spiritual challenges. Getting into nature is very healing for me.

October 1996: I am experiencing an increase in symptoms of depression. Dr. Wallen discontinues the Wellbutrin and starts me on Effexor.

January 1997: I start to experience extreme irritability, a new symptom for me. Dr. Wallen adds the medicine Depakote, which is a mood stabilizer, to my medicine regiment. This month I also participate in the Columbus IPI as the team coordinator. Ross is the facilitator and it's fun to work with him again.

Irrational Medicine

My job is going very well. Over the past year I have hired a very competent staff, a real quality team of people that I enjoy working with. My boss trusts me completely and gives me the budget I need to get the work done. I routinely work the Columbus Basic weekends and develop a close friendship with Susan Estep. Life is good except I just don't seem to be getting the same kick from my medicine that I use to.

January 1997: While working a Basic seminar I meet Linda, a bright, cheerful, fun loving, Italian woman with a smile that can light up a room. I am attracted to her physical beauty and her friendly, outgoing personality. There is something about her, something that mesmerizes me, captivates me. After the seminar we start to see each other on a very frequent basis. Within a few weeks we are in love. I feel "complete" with her. This should be a huge warning sign, but I am getting ready to learn another lesson.

My Body Rebels

March 1997: I contract a mysterious virus that causes huge painful sores to form on the back of my throat. They are so painful that I cannot eat. Despite numerous trips to the emergency room and my family doctor, no one can identify what is causing the sores or any treatment that can help me. I experience overwhelming fatigue and weakness that makes it extremely difficult to perform routine and daily tasks, like getting out of bed, dressing, and eating. The fatigue does not get better with bed rest. For a seven week period I only get out of bed to go to the bathroom and my diet is nothing but liquids. I lose 70 pounds. When I finally return to work it is only for half days. I eventually gain the weight back but I

Irrational Medicine

never return to my previous level of energy. After hundreds of tests and thousands of dollars I am finally diagnosed with Chronic Fatigue Syndrome by a specialist at the Ohio State Medical Center.

When I ask the doctor what is Chronic Fatigue Syndrome his explanation is less than helpful. He says, "It is a noncontagious disease first recognized as a physical illness in the 1980s, but is the subject of a controversy. Even as increasing numbers of people are being diagnosed with the disease, there are still many people inside and outside the health professions who doubt its existence or maintain that it's a psychological ailment. But several years of research have confirmed that it is indeed a physical illness - just one that's not fully understood. The cause is not yet known but research is exploring the possibility that people with the disease may have a dysfunction of the immune and central nervous systems. Some research has suggested that a virus causes it, but this theory has not been proven. However, a viral cause is still suspected because the symptoms of the disease often mimic a viral infection."

I go through the motions of living, but it takes all my effort to get to work and do my job in a cursory way. I feel drained and hopeless. There are no more medical tests or examinations for me to go through, my doctors throw up their hands and send me away because there is nothing they can do for me.

October 1997: My symptoms of depression reoccur. I have an increased need for sleep and poorer energy levels, I feel more irritable, and have very poor motivation, decreased sex drive, increased eating, social withdrawal, and decreased ability to function. Dr. Wallen discontinues the Effexor and starts me back on the Wellbutrin. She keeps me on Depakote.

Irrational Medicine

I continue to do well at work even though my energy level is very low. I love the people and the projects and the financial rewards are great. I convince my boss to pay for my entire staff to attend the Basic seminar. It is so freeing to be able to attend a staff meeting and talk the same language of responsibility and trust. It is also rewarding to see people make long term changes in their lives as a result of going through the training.

My relationship with Linda is always interesting. It has a lot of ups and downs. We are either very happy of very angry with each other. Despite numerous disagreements throughout the relationship I stay with her, telling myself "I just want too much," "I can settle for this, I know I can." Happiness has always been a dream, and I feel unworthy of wanting more than is given to me.

A Scary Experience

January 1998: I don't feel like my medicine is working as well as it could so I change doctors. On my first visit to Dr. Allen he conducts a detailed intake interview and increases the dosage of both the Wellbutrin and the Depakote. He says, "It's a good thing that you are on Depakote because it helps control seizures and Wellbutrin has a fourfold greater tendency to cause seizures than other antidepressants." I am surprised by his comments. No one has ever mentioned anything about possible side effects of my medicine before.

July 1998: I am sitting in my office at work typing on my computer. When I look down all of a sudden and begin to feel very dizzy. Then I get a terrible pain in the center of my chest that feels like an elephant is stepping on me. Then the discomfort

Irrational Medicine

spreads throughout my upper body to my back, neck, and jaw, and I break out in a sweat. I suspect I am having a heart attack, so I call 911 and tell the dispatcher where I am and what is happening. While I wait in my office the pain lessons a little, so I call my children while I wait for the paramedics to arrive. I don't tell them what is happening to me, but I make sure they know how much I love them.

At the emergency room, after my symptoms subside, they admit me to the hospital for further testing. Eventually the cardiologist declares that my heart if fine and that they have no clue why I had such an attack.

Life Continues On

I see Dr. Allen about every two months for approximately 30 minutes each time. During the sessions he asks me how I feel and then discusses either leaving the medicine where it is or increasing one or both dosages. I always leave his office with prescription slips in my hand.

January 2000: Linda and I decide to get married. We can't agree though on the size and cost of the wedding, so we go to a marriage counselor to work it out. In hindsight, seeing a marriage counselor about getting married should have been a red flag. But out of my fearful sense of scarcity I am willing to give in on many things just so I will have someone in my life.

March 2000: I complain to Dr. Allen that I am feeling worse. He says my dosages of the other drugs are very high and he does not want to go any further with those. So he adds the antidepressant Effexor to the Wellbutrin and Depakote.

Irrational Medicine

July 2000: Despite the disapproval of friends and relatives, Linda and I get married. We borrow $10,000 for the wedding and it is a hell of a party. But underneath it all I am angry because I agreed to go into debt for the wedding. My feelings of scarcity and abandonment are so habitual that they influence the way I approach major decisions in my life. I am too willing to compromise who I am in a relationship.

The Letter

November 2000: During the past several months my grandfather's health has been failing. My grandmother calls and says that my grandfather is in the hospital, and he is not doing very well. He has congestive heart failure and fluid is building up in his legs and around his heart. I am getting ready to travel to Las Vegas on business for a week and I want to make damn sure that something doesn't happen to my grandfather before I get a chance to tell him how I feel. So I sit down and write him a letter, because I know I can't say the words to him in person without breaking down in tears. I stop by the hospital on my way to the airport and give him my letter in person.

December 2, 2000
Dear Pappa:
Because we don't know when we will die, we get to think of life as an inexhaustible well. Yet everything happens only a certain amount of times, and a very small number really.
I often wonder how many more times will I remember a certain afternoon of my childhood, some afternoon that's so deeply a part of my being that I can't even conceive of my life without it? Perhaps four or five times more. Perhaps not even that. How many more times will I watch the full moon rise? Perhaps twenty. And yet it all seems limitless.

Irrational Medicine

It's far too easy to take life for granted and assume that we will see the sun rise tomorrow. So I want to tell you some things that have been on my heart for many years.

You have been a huge influence in my life. Some of my fondest memories of my childhood are of the times I have spent with you. I vividly remember when you would play baseball with me in the backyard. I remember that when I outgrew the toy glove I played with you would use it. I remember when you gave me and Garry a quarter. We were both surprised and elated because we usually had to go to Mamma for money. Another time you gave me a sip of your beer even though Mamma had yelled at you for doing it.

Christmas at your house was always very special. Garry and I would try to go to sleep in the "twin beds" but were too excited. Also going on vacations with you were exciting. There are too many memories for me to list here but I want you to know that Garry and I loved to spend time with you and Mamma.

While you have never been a person that expresses feelings very openly I have always known that you loved me. This was evident many years ago when I saw that you carried my high school picture in your wallet. I am extremely grateful to God that you are my grandfather. Naming my first born son after you was a way of demonstrating my gratitude for all you have meant to me and for the tremendous amount of respect I have for you as a man.

There is a principle of alchemy that states: things which have once been in contact with each other continue to act on each other at a distance even after the physical contact has been severed. This is true for our relationship as well. You will continue to impact my life and the life of my children in ways that you will never know. Thank you for all you have done for me.

There once was a dying King who called his wise men together and instructed them to come up with an inscription for his tombstone. His instructions were that the inscription should be good for a thousand years and after that till the end of the world. It was to be something so true that no matter what happened it would stand. Something that no matter who spit on it or laughed at it there it would stand and nothing would change it. They thought for quite some time and finally found the answer. Five simple words: THIS TOO SHALL PASS AWAY.

Irrational Medicine

> *Indeed, death is not the final answer. In Romans 6:23 the Bible tells us "For the wages of sin is death, but for the gift of God is eternal life in Christ Jesus our Lord."*
> *I love you and I will see you and Garry on the other side.*
> Jeff

December 15, 2000: My grandfather has been transferred to a nursing home. My grandfather has been a key part of my life and I am so sad to see him deteriorate like this. He has always been there for me when I needed help. He hates it in the nursing home and begs to go home to die. Finally after Christmas my grandmother and dad take him home.

January 18, 2001: I return to Dr. Allen and complain of anxiety and irritability. After the typical 15 minute question and answer session, he adds the anti-anxiety drug Buspar to the Effexor, Wellbutrin, and Depakote I am already taking.

January 26, 2001: It is Thursday night of the Basic seminar in Columbus, and I am scheduled to work it. While getting ready to leave the house, the telephone rings. It is my grandmother, she says, "Your grandfather is wondering why you haven't been by lately. He really wants to see you." Something inside me says to go see him so I say, "I am working this weekend but I will come by for a few hours Saturday morning." I figure that's a slow time for what I have to do during the seminar, and I can probably get away with not being there for a few hours.

January 28, 2001 (Saturday): I drive 72 miles from Columbus to Dayton to see my grandfather. I walk in the house, kiss my grandmother hello and go into the family room where my grandfather is lying in a hospital bed. As I walk to the bed I see the family pictures on the walls and the curtains covering the patio door are open. It is a beautiful sunny but cold

Irrational Medicine

day. I say, "Hi, Pappa." He is half asleep but knows who I am and responds, "Hey, Buddy Boy." It is so hard for me to see this man who has been so strong and independent all his life lying in a bed he can't even get out of on his own. He eats a Popsicle because his throat is dry. I sit next to his bed for 3 hours while he goes in and out of consciousness.

Then it is time to go because I promised the team that I will be back by 1:00 p.m. I touch my grandfather's arm, lean over and kiss him on the forehead and say, "I love you." He says, "I love you too," without opening his eyes.

I cry for most of the trip home, thinking that maybe this is the last time I will see him alive. When I return to the seminar I tell Susan what happened. She says that she has read how people can put off their passing in order to see those they love just one more time.

At 7:00 p.m. I get a phone call on my cell phone from Dad. He says, "After you left this morning your grandfather went into a comatose state and started breathing very heavily. This might be it. I suggest that you come to the house." I don't hesitate and I tell the seminar leader what is happening and that I must leave. I get into my Ford Explorer and begin to drive west toward Dayton to make that 72 mile trip again.

As I drive I call Linda to tell her what is going on. She has some of her friends over for a party since I am working the Basic all weekend. I explain that I have just left the seminar and am heading for Dayton because it looks like this might be my grandfather's passing. Several minutes later my dad calls and says not to hurry that because my grandfather just died a few minutes ago.

I am devastated. Even though I knew it was

Irrational Medicine

inevitable, it still saddens me to lose such a wonderful man in my life.

I call Linda back to tell her that he is dead. She says to call her when I get to Dayton. About 30 minutes later after crying a terrible cry I call my ex-wife Tina so she can tell the boys that their great-grandfather has gone on to be with God. Tina asks if I want her to bring the boys to my grandmother's house. This catches me by surprise. Then it dawns on me; I have been in so much sorrow that I have not stopped to realize that Linda is not with me, nor did she even bother to ask if I want her to be with me. I am going through one of the worst nights of my life because of the passing of one of the most important people in my life and my wife is at home partying with her friends.

I tell Tina that it isn't necessary to bring the boys up tonight because it is so late. But she can bring them up in the morning. I hang up the phone and stare straight ahead at the highway.

When I arrive at my grandparents' house my dad and stepmother are there waiting for me. The funeral home has already picked up my grandfather's body. The first question my dad asks is where is Linda? All of the thoughts and disappointments I had just lived through for the past hour came tearing through my mind. I make up some bullshit excuse that my dad doesn't seem to believe, which is not surprising since I didn't believe it myself. It is very apparent that I am not the only one who thinks a wife should be with her husband during such a time.

February 2001: During my office visit with Dr. Allen, I request that the he discontinue the Effexor. It is causing me to experience less than adequate erections and premature ejaculation.

Irrational Medicine

Later I go back to the marriage counselor by myself because I want to talk to about how Linda treated me the night my grandfather passed away. After several minutes of my ranting and raving, the counselor asks me if anyone has ever suggested that I might have Attention Deficit Disorder (ADD). I confess that I don't even know what ADD is. She gives me a 10 question quiz that suggests that I have ADD. Then she refers me to a specialist for further testing and diagnosis.

Chapter 6

A Second Wound

Each transformation is going to be painful because the old has to be left for the new.
- OSHO

March 2001: I go to a psychiatrist who specializes in the diagnosis of ADD. She starts the visit with an interview and takes a detailed history of my symptoms. Then she administers a 14 part test she says will measure my cognitive performance in several key areas including word analysis and spatial reasoning. Some test sections are questions only, other parts involve drawings, other parts are more like puzzles where I move blocks around to match a picture. Some parts are timed, some are not. She grills me on my math skills, knowledge of history, geography, and English. I feel as though she is testing my intelligence rather than my attention. The whole process takes four hours to complete.

Five days later I return to get the results. The doctor starts the meeting by blurting out: "You not only have ADD but it is so severe that if you didn't have such a high IQ, you would be flipping hamburgers for a living." I am shocked by such a blunt announcement. She goes on to explain: "You behave in ways that demonstrate poor attention, distractibility, poor self control, impulsivity, excessive activity, also known as hyperactivity, and distractibility, which can be seen as the tendency to

Irrational Medicine

constantly monitor one's environment for prey opportunities, or to avoid becoming prey." I ask, "How did you determine this?" She says, "I reviewed the pattern of scores between the subsets of the IQ test to determine attention problems. This information is then considered with the results of the clinical interview to determine the nature of an attention problem if one is present." I say, "So the testing you conducted was nothing more than an IQ test?" She says, "That's right. IQ is not associated with ADD, but my evaluation is not based on your answers but on your behavior during the test. I observed your body language, as well as your ability or inability to concentrate. Any kind of written test could have been used instead of an IQ test. Then I apply the criteria from the Diagnostics and Statistics Manual (DSM) to make my final determination."

She pulls out the DSM and reviews the symptoms with me.

- Often fidgets with hands or feet or squirms in seat.
- Often leaves seat in classroom or in other situations in which remaining seated is expected.
- Often runs about or climbs excessively in situations in which it is inappropriate (in adolescents or adults, may be limited to subjective feelings of restlessness).
- Often has difficulty playing or engaging in leisure activities quietly.
- Is often "on the go" or often acts as if "driven by a motor."
- Often talks excessively.
- Often blurts out answers before questions have been completed.
- Often has difficulty waiting turn.

Irrational Medicine

- Often interrupts or intrudes on others (e.g., butts into conversations or games).

    Basically by using the DSM, a person can be diagnosed as having ADD simply on the basis that he or she exhibits six or more of the listed symptoms for at least six months, to a degree that is maladaptive and impairs functioning.

    With the DSM, the psychiatrist no longer needs to spend tedious hours searching for the reasons why a patient suffers from anxiety, agitation or other symptoms. They simply have to identify a sufficient number of symptoms to shoehorn the patient into a "diagnostic" category. Psychiatrists use DSM as a substitute for an actual diagnosis.

    (One thing the doctor fails to consider is that drug induced agitation looks very much like ADD. Antidepressants commonly cause a stimulant like effect called akathisia - the inability to sit or stand still, which happens to be a common symptom of ADD. The side effects of the antidepressants I am taking can easily account for almost every one of the diagnostic criteria for ADD.)

    I take my diagnosis, go home and experience some level of relief because my problem has been diagnosed a medical condition rather than some kind of moral or emotional failure.

A Teacher Shows Up

    Now that I have a diagnosis I want to know more about ADD. The next morning at 9:00 a.m. I open the phone book and start calling doctors offices listed with the specialty of ADD support. After several calls I find a doctor who has a cancellation for an 11:00 a.m. appointment that very morning. I take the

Irrational Medicine

appointment and in a little while I am sitting in front of Dr. Leisa Fleetwood.

Our first session is pretty standard. She is a psychologist, a petite blonde woman with a pleasant smile and a delightfully playful manner about her. I explain my recent diagnosis and some of the things that are going on in my life. Since it's our first meeting we don't get into a lot of details, but for some reason I feel very comfortable with her, like I know her from somewhere. I can sense that she is more than a typical doctor.

A few days later I have another appointment with Dr. Allen and I tell him about the results of my ADD test. He adds the medicine Concerta, a longer-acting form of Ritalin, to my Buspar, Wellbutrin, and Depakote. I take the prescription with the anticipation that this is the medicine I have been needing to get better. I have lost confidence in my ability to cope without medication.

Ritalin

Ritalin belongs to the class of drugs known as stimulants and is closely related to amphetamines – it is essentially a form of speed. In 1971, Ritalin joined morphine, opium, and barbiturates in Schedule 2 of the Controlled Substances Act due to its very high potential for abuse. Studies indicate that Ritalin has very similar effects on the brain as amphetamine, methamphetamines, and cocaine. This includes impairment of emotional responsiveness and mental functions. Since Ritalin is a stimulant it can produce the very symptoms it is supposed to control, hyperactivity, impulsively, and inattention. The United States produces and uses 90 percent of the world's Ritalin.

Irrational Medicine

My first day taking the Ritalin produces a very strange and unusual reaction. I have always had a poor sense of smell but for some reason after taking the Ritalin I can smell a lot more than usual. This only lasts a few days and never occurs again. The biggest difference I notice right away is an increase in my energy level. I also experience feelings of euphoria, a sense of power, alertness, excitement, heightened clarity, and an ability to get by with less than six hours of sleep. It is very similar to the effect that antidepressants use to have on me when I first started taking them. I feel good for the first time in years.

Dr. Fleetwood and I meet weekly. I look forward to our time together because she is different from any therapist or doctor I have ever known. Not only do we discuss ADD but we talk about my relationship with Linda and eventually we begin to discuss metaphysics. Dr. Fleetwood talks to me about energy systems of the body and the need for balance in my life. She even gives me a tutoring session on tarot cards because I question why bad things keep happening to me. She teaches me that our physical bodies are containers for our consciousness that allow us to interact strongly with objects and people in the physical world. In reality our consciousness reaches beyond the brain and the physical body to the level of our spiritual anatomy and our extended multidimensional energy fields. At first I find her entertaining because I don't believe all of this new age stuff. But after several conversations where she says things to me that only my family members would have been aware of I start to think she knows what she is talking about.

We discuss the Human Potential movement and how I am actually on a quest to become all I am capable of being. We talk about process, philosophy,

Irrational Medicine

and the logic of combining Zen and metaphysics with self-awareness and self-acceptance. Dr. Fleetwood does not reinforce my feelings of helplessness and indecision. Instead all of her counsel aims to inspire me with the capacity to take charge of my own life. She is very empathic and caring – she brings a compassionate spirit to the therapy. Instead of emphasizing my "mental illness" she starts teaching me how to draw on my own human potential and natural assets. She encourages me to reestablish the "locus of control" within myself and strengthens my sense of personal autonomy, self-understanding, and decision making.

May 2001: I start a new job with a Fortune 500 company in Columbus. They are the world's largest distributor of pharmaceutical drugs - a fact I would later come to find thoroughly ironic.

Married Life

Linda and I go through the motions of being married but we can't communicate. I am very quick to anger and when she asks anything of me I stonewall her. When she seeks contact and offers to talk, I just scowl, watch television, or pretend to sleep, waiting for the storm to blow over. Linda begins to talk louder and louder and eventually starts shouting. After months of criticism, of attacks and counterattacks, I mentally withdraw and emotionally abandon the marriage. I physically stay with Linda because I have convinced myself how few good women there are out there. I have resigned myself to a life where love and joy will never come in abundance.

Dr. Fleetwood says, "Every marriage faces a crisis when one or both partners realize the spouse is not able to help solve one's own neurotic problems.

Irrational Medicine

The original attraction between future spouses is that each sees the other as a way of solving his or her own self-esteem issues. Who you fall in love with is determined by your particular psychological needs at the time you enter a relationship. And those needs will have to get addressed somehow in the relationship or it will never work" I say, "So that's why I have been willing to compromise who I am just to be with Linda? I am not yet a complete person. I rely on her hope her enthusiasm to be in the relationship." Dr. Fleetwood says, "What attracted you to each other was a defense – you saw her cheerful outgoing attitude as something missing from your life. She saw you as the strong silent type, and she needed strength. What you didn't realize is that her cheerfulness hid some sort of lack of self esteem, and she didn't realize that your silence came from anxiety rather than strength. What once were virtues are now defects. The things that once attracted you to each other now seem to push you apart. Instead of loving those qualities, you each hate them. You de-idealize each other; that initial stage of being 'in love' is gone."

In another session Dr. Fleetwood teaches me that spirituality is about expansion and growth. It is about love, truth, goodness, beauty, giving, and caring. It's about wholeness and completion. It is our ultimate human need. It's critical to make a clear distinction between spirituality and religion. She says, "Spirituality is based on direct experiences of other realities. It does not necessarily require a special place or a special person mediating contact with the divine. Spirituality involves a special relationship between the individual and the cosmos and is in essence a personal and private affair."

Dr. Fleetwood introduces me to a form of meditation she calls Flow. Prior to each session she

Irrational Medicine

has me write down what my intention is for the meditation. Then she facilitates the session with that intention. I usually lie on a table or recline in an easy chair. She touches my head and meditates. After a few minutes I can feel an energy pulsating through my body. It is flowing from my feet to my head like a river. Dr. Fleetwood says "The healing comes from the collective unconscious and it is guided by an inner intelligence that surpasses that of any individual therapist. My task is simply to offer a safe environment that helps you get into a trance, and support you unconditionally with full trust, which allows the spontaneous unfolding of the process. Healing and resolution often occur in ways that transcend rational understanding. In this form of therapy, I am not the doer, merely a sympathetic supporter and co adventurer." I don't know if I am making up the experience of each session or what, but afterwards I always feel better so I keep doing it. After each session we talk about what I felt and what she experienced during the meditation. She says, "You will eventually be capable of doing this by yourself, I am just facilitating the sessions until you grow into self sufficiency. You should investigate energy work on your own. There are Reiki classes held around town. It would be a good idea for you to go to one."

As our weekly sessions continue Dr. Fleetwood warns me: "Most men are task oriented and they like to know when the job is done, but the milestones of healing are not always easy to distinguish. You must have faith. Faith in yourself is the strongest medicine you have for fighting the tendency to give up too early. You have to believe in your ability to heal and become the type of person you want to be. You are struggling with the suppression of your feminine side. You actually fear your feminine side, so you try to control

Irrational Medicine

it. Since that is what you focus on, you attract women that are uncontrollable like Linda. You have denied your feelings, your sense of vulnerability, your loneliness, your need for companionship and tender love. The feminine side will allow you to be more intimately involved with your children, more emotional and more in touch with your feelings. You will be less afraid to seem vulnerable. Linda represents the feminine traits in you that you most admire. You now need to start to focus on what you want - start to create your own experience."

At home I am dying in pieces. I dread coming home at night. Linda and I talk at the table on the most superficial "how was your day" level. I avoid going to bed till after she is asleep. I am depressed and angry whenever I am around her. And yet making the move to pick up and go feels like walking into an abyss and seems more depressing than staying. My fear of closeness is so great that I defend against it by closing off, by coldness, by keeping her at such a distance that all of her own needs for intimacy and sharing are denied. These kinds of frustrations and deprivations have become so chronic and pervasive that much of the joy and love has been drained out of our relationship.

November 21, 2001: During my session with Dr. Fleetwood I say, "I am in a constant state of turmoil in my relationship with Linda, and I fear that things will only get worse. As a matter of fact my life has been in turmoil the entire time we have known each other. I have never had the nerve to walk away from her and forget her. Every logical bone in my body says run, but I just don't want to deal with not having her around." Dr. Fleetwood says, "Obviously you still have lessons to learn, and Linda is here to help you do so. One of the ways we work out our issues is in relationships."

I ask, "Is it possible to reach a point where you have "worked out" as much as you're going to get and it is time to move on to the next one?" Dr. Fleetwood replies, "Absolutely. But right now you need to decide if you want to be married or not. You are neither in the game or out of it. You must decide." I say, "It would be easy to make a decision about the relationship if she just had an affair. I wouldn't have to struggle with a decision then it would be an automatic end to the relationship" Little did I realize that the Universe was about to help me make a decision.

Betrayal and Divorce - Again

The next day is Thanksgiving, and I don't see much of Linda because she goes to her mother's house to help prepare dinner for her family. The day after that is Friday and I don't see her at all because she is shopping with her friends and that evening she has to work at the bingo hall.

November 24, 2001: It's 4:30 am Saturday morning and I am in bed sleeping. Linda comes home four hours after getting off of work at the bingo hall. After she comes to bed I lie there unable to sleep, tossing and turning. I have a nagging feeling, a little voice tells me to check her cell phone. I have never done that before, but this voice won't leave me alone. I quietly slip out of bed go downstairs and find her cell phone on the charging stand. I look at the outbound call logs. They show that she made calls to someone named Eric at 10:30 p.m., 11:20 p.m., 12:00 a.m. and 1:00 a.m., that morning. I am very suspicious because every other entry in the log includes a first

Irrational Medicine

and last name. Eric is the only one without a last name.

By now it's 5:30 a.m. I go back upstairs and confront her with what I have found. I want to know why she is home so late, and who is Eric? She tells me they are friends. She works with him at the bingo hall. He has been having trouble with his wife, and they just get together to talk. He tells her about how bad he has it at home, and she tells him what's happening in our marriage. But I can see on her face that there is much more to the story.

Something overwhelming boils inside of me and I decide in that instant that this marriage is over. I do not what someone in my life who can betray me. I decide that I am not going to waste any more time trying to work on the marriage. I learned from my first marriage that for a woman to cheat on her husband she has to disengage from the relationship, to fall out of love with him. That's a huge hole to work out of and I am not willing to waste any time on the effort. Even if Linda hasn't physically done anything, which I seriously doubt knowing her, she has emotionally cheated on me by seeking comfort with another man.

I tell Linda to get out of my house. She calls her family and friends who come over and help her pack. By 10:30 a.m. Saturday morning Linda is gone, the marriage is over.

Things Will Be Different

I make a firm resolution with myself that this time I am not going to have an emotional breakdown like I did at the end of my first marriage. I have come too far and learned too much to let that happen. I contact Dr. Fleetwood and talk with her about what

Irrational Medicine

has happened. She meets me in the office for a Flow meditation that afternoon.

My intent for the Flow meditation is for assistance in finding my self-love and acceptance inside and support in coming to peace in my relationship with myself and others. I am asking that I evolve with ease and joy for the highest good of all.

After the meditation Dr. Fleetwood and I debrief as usual. I say, "I saw many faces of people I don't know. They were all in black and white and there were a lot them one after another. When I came out of the meditation the thought: I can't give away something I don't have, popped into my mind."

Dr. Fleetwood says, "It was the most humbling experience I have ever had. It felt deep and heavy. I saw a tree that lost its structure and sank into the soil. Then it waited and rebuilt itself from a different perspective. I felt an incredible amount of grace. Your rebuilding is completely supported and right timing. Layer after layer after layer spun around the form of you, killing the ego; letting go of control. I saw you evolving toward true presence, authentic power."

Considering what I went through this morning I feel pretty good right now.

Energy Medicine

I remember meeting a lady by the name of Tere Banks while working at a Basic seminar. She told me about Reiki, an ancient Japanese healing method that uses the laying on of hands to heal. She is a Reiki Master and practices it. I don't know whether I believe in it or not but I am so determined not to crash again that I am willing to try anything to keep from having a breakdown. So I call Tere and make an appointment.

She starts our session by describing her work.

Irrational Medicine

"In addition to our physical bodies there is another form of energy important to human health which is spiritual energy. Spiritual energy flows into the cells and organs of the physical body through various forms and pathways. One pathway is through the unique system of seven major energy centers known as chakras. Chakras are specialized energy centers throughout the body where a unique form of subtle life energy is absorbed and distributed to the cells, organs, and body tissues. However, the flow of this energy, also known as prana, through our chakras is strongly affected by our personality and our emotions, as well as our state of spiritual development. Each chakra is linked to a different region of the body. Seven main chakras exist in the body, along with many other minor chakra centers and could actually be considered emotional and spiritual energy processors

    Throughout our lifetime each of the chakras processes and remembers different emotional events and traumas that affect us. We seem to store specific types of emotional memories in each center. Perhaps this is one of the reasons we remember things not only with our brains but with our bodies as well. This might also explain why different types of emotional distress seem to affect one part of the body differently than another. The flow of life energy to each of the seven charkas and their associated body regions is strongly affected by the way we process emotional and spiritual issues in our lives. When someone has a chronic problem in dealing with emotional and spiritual issues associated with a particular chakra, the resulting constriction of life energy flow to that part of the body can sometimes manifest as a disease or some other health challenge.

    The chakras also form a major part of our link

Irrational Medicine

with our soul; so when someone's chakras are blocked, it may be because there are difficulties with psychological and spiritual issues to which they are not giving adequate attention. Chakra linked issues can be tied to the functionality of our relationships with ourselves, family members, loved ones, and even co-workers. Our attitudes and emotional reactions play an important role in whether we will be vibrantly healthy or chronically ill. Where an illness occurs in the body is often an indicator of which particular psychospiritual issues a person needs to direct attention to in order to achieve inner rebalancing and a recovery of health.

    The first or root chakra is our connection to the earth, the energy center where concerns over survival and personal safety are processed. For example, someone who feels threatened and unsafe in the world may eventually develop an associated balance in the root center. The second chakra is connected with our personal and working relationships with others. The third, also known as the solar plexus chakra, is affected by the way we deal with the issues surrounding our personal power and our self-esteem.

    The fourth, also known as the heart chakra, is one of the most critical because this is where the issues surrounding love and nurturance most strongly affect us. Whether or not we consider ourselves to be "lovable" and chronic difficulties in expressing love toward others may eventually contribute to physical problems affecting the heart and lungs, as well as to immunity related disorders making us more susceptible to infections and other serious health problems.

    The fifth center, also known as the throat chakra, is associated with communication of thoughts, opinions, and ideas. The throat chakra is

Irrational Medicine

also linked with issues surrounding the expression of our will. People who are always afraid to speak their minds or to voice their ideas and concerns can sometimes develop imbalances in their fifth emotional-energy center, resulting in chronic throat problems, recurrent laryngitis, or even thyroid disease.

    The sixth or brow chakra is associated with various aspects of mental activities and the intellect. Whether or not we have a clear vision of where we are headed and what we are doing with our lives directly influences energy flow through the brow chakra. The seventh, or crown chakra is our connection to God or the Universe. Here resides our sense of purpose in life as well as our sense of spiritual connection with God. The seventh chakra is intimately related to our search for purpose and meaning in life, especially with regard to our link with the divine."

    Tere then does a 45 minute Reiki treatment on me. I can feel the sensation of heat at various places on my body as she moves her hands over me. Throughout the session Tere comments on what comes to her as visions. She says, "If there is any doubt that Linda and you are through, you can put it out of your mind. The relationship is definitely over. You have an incredible amount of anger that you need to get out somehow. You learned most of your expectations about relationships from your mother. Because of what you are going through with Linda you will have the opportunity to make tremendous strides toward spirituality. In March you will not recognize yourself."

    After the session Tere tells me what she saw, "Your crown is very closed. Energy can't get out the top of your head. Your third eye is in great shape but your throat is out of shape. You have a lot to say but

Irrational Medicine

you are holding it in. Your solar plexus is large and filled with fear. Your core beliefs are very small.

Later that evening at home I am stricken by grief and I fall to my knees and pray to God that "Thy will be done." I am so tired of swimming upstream and I am just going to trust that everything will work out for the best. I continue to spend a tremendous amount of time in meditation and prayer. I read every self help book I can get my hands on. I also start taking Bach Flower remedies, a unique form of vibrational medicine that has become increasingly popular over the last sixty years. And I start seeing an acupuncturist.

December 5 2001: Today Dr. Fleetwood starts our session with a tarot reading. It shows that the reason I am going through another divorce is to raise my consciousness. I mention my concern about taking another fall like I did in 1995. She says, "That is not possible because you are too advanced mentally and emotionally. You must remember that the problems in your relationship were only symptoms. The real problem is your lack of self-love, confidence, and knowing that you are fine just the way you are. You are learning all of these things. You will survive this and you will be a better person for having gone through it."

Later that night as I sit in my bedroom my meditation is very deep and tremendously peaceful. A vision of a beautiful white light floods my mind. Then I hear a powerful strong voice in my right ear say "Jeff." I get the feeling that who or whatever this is it does not mean me any harm. They simply want me to know they are with me. I continue meditating for several minutes.

December 12, 2001: I complain to Dr. Fleetwood about my chronic fatigue, depression, ADD,

Irrational Medicine

crippling shyness, low self-esteem, unfulfilled dreams, jealousy, possessiveness, lack of abundance, lack of joy, too much anger, and fear. She says, "Just keep doing what you're doing. You are working through the fear and pain."

December 16, 2001: Jordan, my youngest son, and I visit the Unity church in Columbus. It is fun to be in a place where fire and brimstone isn't shoved down your throat. Instead they keep focusing on love and a universal power. I pray for God to guide me toward my next step with ease and joy. Afterwards I get a strong urge to go to the Barnes and Noble at the Lennox Town Center mall. I have no desire to buy another book, but I go any way. I am walking down the audio book aisle and right at eye level in a pink box was a tape set called "The Heart of the Soul; Emotional Awareness." Of course with a title like that and what I am going through I have to buy it.

I Discover Energy Work

December 21, 2001: I take Dr. Fleetwood's advice and enroll in a Reiki class. The day starts with an introduction to Reiki principles of healing. Then several hours of training and finally an attunement from a Reiki Master. To wrap up the day, all the new students and several Reiki Masters get together and practice on one another.

This all seems so far out to me but I go along with it. I am willing to try anything and then I can be the judge as to whether or not it works.

When it's my turn to use Reiki there is a lady on the table. I hold my hands about six inches above her body and start to move them from her head to her feet. As I cross her stomach I feel a strong tingling sensation in both of my hands. After I pass over her

Irrational Medicine

stomach the tingling stops. I repeat the movement and once again the tingling starts as I move over her stomach. It is the weirdest thing I have ever experienced. It's like turning on a light switch. When my hands are over her stomach I feel the tingling, when they're not I don't.

One of the Reiki Masters is at my table and I tell her what is happening. She says, "That is not unusual. A healer can usually feel a cycle of sensations. You may feel sensations of heat, cold, water flowing, vibrating, trembling, magnetism, static electricity, tingling, color, sound or in extremely rare cases pain moving through your hands. The person receiving the healing may experience the same things or different ones, or she may feel nothing." After my turn to practice on my fellow student she tells me that she has been battling cancer, right in the area where I could feel the tingling in my hands..

Then it's my turn to get on the table. The Reiki Master at my table calls over one of the other Reiki Masters. Before it is all over I am on the table for 75 minutes with up to five people at a time working on me. They say things such as, my entire left side (my emotional side) is shut down, and my right side is way overbuilt (extremely powerful) to compensate for it. I also have had a major loss of someone significant to me when I was younger. They say that within the last two months I have lost a family. (This probably refers to Linda's family since we are now split.) They also say that my body carries the memory of a horrible death (at a minimum a beheading and probably even more) from a past life. At the end, they tell me that my left side has opened up and the energy is quivering. It's like a muscle that hasn't been used for some time, and it will quiver until it gets use to working again.

Irrational Medicine

They hold a pendant over my heart and it moves in big circles counterclockwise all by itself. One of the masters is from OSU and she comments "Usually people can't hide from me but you are able to." I have no idea what to make of that comment.

The class instructor gets involved and does some cranial sacral work on me. One lady uses a tuning fork. She says it is to generate a certain sound that my body needs to hear. Someone else uses stones and oils. I feel as if I am at a new age science fair. I am not sure what to make of all the things they are doing to me but at a minimum it is entertaining. At the end of the day when I leave I feel pretty good. I feel lighter and more cheerful than when the day started.

When I get home I become curious about my new skill so I sit down in the living room and call my dog over. I turn him around so his back is facing me and he is looking in the other direction. I hold my hands about six inches above his back. As soon as I silently invoke the Reiki command he turns his head and looks at me. He starts to squirm and then it seems like he becomes uncomfortable and scampers away. It certainly seems as if he can sense something when I "treat" him. I try it several more times throughout the evening and each time he responds when I silently invoke the Reiki command. I begin to believe this stuff is for real.

December 26, 2001: Dr. Fleetwood warns me that I tend to view everything in terms of "good or bad" and "win or lose," because that's the way I was brought up. She also counsels me that we are here on the earth school to learn lessons. The same lessons will be presented to us over and over until we learn them. So I must take advantage of the current situation to learn my lesson.

Irrational Medicine

January 3, 2002: Dr. Fleetwood says, "If something hurts you do not have to allow it. You can choose to draw the line at anything that causes you pain." I say, "So when Linda went out bar hopping with her friends I could say that was unacceptable?" Dr. Fleetwood, "You have every right to say that it is unacceptable and you will not tolerate it. Now it may have meant the end of your relationship, because she also has the right to say what is and isn't acceptable to her. We all have the right to determine what behaviors we will allow in our lives." These words are a big relief because I can stop looking for the magic relationship book with the "rules" in it. All I have to do is determine whether or not I am comfortable with a situation. She says, "Just remember that clarity comes from thoughts (your head) backed by emotions (your heart)."

January 6, 2002: During a Reiki session Tere sees a woman by the name of either Linda or Lila, with brown hair and green eyes. She thinks she may be an angel. She also notices a strong tension, quivering energy in my left shoulder. She says that I am on the verge of knowing my truth, setting my beliefs (right now they are a blank slate), and giving my gifts, that my chakras are in good shape, and that my throat is now capable of speaking my truth and my heart will guide my words. In the past I withheld my true words to accommodate others.

January 10, 2002: Dr. Fleetwood can sense a change in my energy, that I have made a major shift. She speculates that my Reiki training has helped to open up my energy field and suggests that I practice it on anything and everything.

She observes that I am also answering my own questions now. I routinely share my journal pages with Dr. Fleetwood so she can see what is happening

Irrational Medicine

inside my mind. She says, "Your journals show swings in emotion, while staying on an even keel as an observer. You are feeling your emotions, but you are not letting them run your life. It's probably time for you to form new beliefs." This strikes me as odd because that's what Tere referred to in our Reiki session.

Chapter 7

Where Your Wound Is, That's Where Your Genius Is

The greatest thing in the world is to know how to belong to ourselves.
- Michel De Montaigne

January 14, 2002: During a weekly session with Dr. Fleetwood she loans me a copy of the book *King, Warrior, Magician, Lover: Rediscovering the Archetypes of the Mature Masculine,* by Robert Moore and Douglas Gillette. The content of the book fascinates me. It begins with a short introduction on the difference between immature boy psychology and mature man psychology and some of their manifestations. Then mythology and Jungian psychology are used to explain and highlight the benevolent King, the courageous and disciplined Warrior, the capable and knowledgeable Magician, and the connected and loyal Lover. For each, the authors explain and differentiate between their full expression and their "shadow" (i.e. dysfunctional) forms that provide a guide for what really needs repair within the psyche. Arguing that mature masculinity is not abusive or domineering, but generative, creative, and empowering of the self and others, Moore and Gillette provide a Jungian introduction to the psychological foundations of a mature, authentic, and revitalized masculinity.

Irrational Medicine

By far the most intriguing thought in the book for me is the authors assertion that the problem with this world and men is that there is an overwhelming dominance of boyish, immature masculinity and hardly any mature, male masculinity. To paraphrase the author: The world is full of boys pretending to be men.

When I finish this book I have such a thirst for more of this type of information that I do a search for similar books on Amazon.com. The top hit reveals a book called *The Way of the Superior Man* by David Deida, which I immediately order for overnight delivery.

The Way of The Superior Man arrives the next afternoon and I read it in three days. The book takes me on a powerful journey into the heart of the contemporary masculine experience. Deida has a way of cutting through the bullshit and the political correctness and getting right to the point. With uncommon honesty, he explores the most challenging and important issues in men's lives. He covers everything from work and career, to dealing with sex, women, and love, to finding purpose in an increasingly superficial world. What emerges is a wholly revolutionary look at what it means to be a man in today's world, as well as an astonishingly practical guidebook to living a masculine life of integrity, authenticity, and freedom.

The book reveals how a man can live a life of fulfillment without compromise by relaxing into the truth of his very being, discovering his deepest vision, and giving his gifts without holding anything back. Concerning relationships, Deida gives examples and explanations that ring true as to why things happen the way they do and solutions to those problems that feel true to me. The book allows me to understand my

Irrational Medicine

ex-wives, as though someone has just taken a blindfold off. This book rocks my world to its very foundation and changes my view of life at the most profound possible level. The message of the book seems to be - get off your ass and start making something special of your life and your relationships.

I immediately go to Deida's web site and order every book he has written and every audio tape he has produced. Over the next few days I listen to the tapes in the car to and from work and read all his books. My soul has such a thirst for this knowledge that I soak the material up like a sponge. In one of the books a paragraph refers to the need for men to have more companionship with other men and talks about the work of an organization called The ManKind Project. I feel compelled to check out their web site at MKP.org.

God Answers

January 21, 2002: On the MKP website is a description of a training called The New Warrior Training Adventure. It describes the training in the following manner:

> *The ManKind Project® offers trainings which support men in developing lives of integrity, accountability, and connection to feeling. Our trainings challenge men to develop their abilities as leaders, fathers, and elders as ways of offering their deepest gifts in service to the world.*
>
> *The ManKind Project's New Warrior Training Adventure™ is an intense, transformative men's initiation which invites men to forge a deep conscious connection between head and heart.*

Irrational Medicine

The NWTA offers men a powerful, challenging opportunity to look at all aspects of their lives in a richly supportive environment.

As I read the description I hear a little voice say "This is what you have been waiting for all your life" and I know without a doubt that I must attend the training. I feel so strongly that I have been led to this site by a force beyond my control. The next morning I call the Chicago office and find out that there is a training at Phantom Lake, Wisconsin in four days. It starts Friday evening and lasts until Sunday afternoon. I pay the tuition via a credit card and give them all my registration information, no questions asked.

As soon as I hang up the phone I start to cry. I am afraid because I have no idea what to expect but I also know at a deep level that my life is about to change, again. I long to uncover my life's true purpose, embrace fear as an ally, and express my unique sacred gifts with others. I am looking forward to this weekend.

At The Camp

January 24, 2002: After ten hours on the road I arrive at the camp in Wisconsin. It is so cold that the lake surrounding the camp is frozen solid.

I spend the next three days working through the major mental, emotional and spiritual issues in my life. The New Warrior weekend is an initiation training intended to highlight the drama of a man's life and expose it to an intensive mirroring. For me, it turns out to be an experience in which shame has little chance to escape exposure. It is designed to reinstitute an initiation into manhood that male elders

Irrational Medicine

in our culture have long neglected. Traditional rituals from several cultures are combined creatively with the modern. There are numerous experiential exercises designed to teach many different lessons. As in traditional initiation, men are tested physically, emotionally, and spiritually. Several times throughout the weekend I am overwhelmed by helplessness and fear, but I thoroughly understood my urgent need for finding a meaningful way of life, so each time I find within myself deep reserves of strength that I hardly knew existed.

    The staff of the weekend uses Jungian archetypes, strong spiritual containers, a commitment to integrity, active listening, and intuitively inspired processes to support the men going through the weekend, in uncovering, confronting, and transforming the underlying emotional landscape of our lives. For me it specifically means reclaiming the parts of me that I abandoned as a child or young man in my desire to fit in and gain approval. And it means dealing with the part of me that is still a hurt, wounded, scared little boy - except now the boy is trapped in my adult body.

    The processes during the weekend allow me to address my personal issues in ways I have not been able to in therapy. I enter into the emotional, physical, and spiritual experience of being present and intentional with other men, and emerge deeply touched, excited and somehow changed. The initiation processes ground me in honest acceptance and responsibility for myself. From this new viewpoint, I learn to pursue my goals by taking action that is responsible rather than reactive to others. I become receptive, rather than reactive to other people. For the first time I am able to say I need, I hurt, and I can't to myself and others instead of hiding behind a macho

Irrational Medicine

or a nice guy persona.

The weekend shows me how to meet my needs with other men. It helps me develop a remarkable new ability to be emotionally present and communicate with people. The leaders redefine the standards for what a man is. I am taught that a real man does the hard work of finding, naming, and owning his own feelings. I am challenged to be a man who acts with integrity among other men, directed from within by my own sense of mission. I see that a man needs other men in his life, and needs to be loved by other men. I discover new possibilities for being a good son and father.

Discoveries About Myself

As the weekend progresses I am being shown who I am with incredible speed and intensity. I am given much grace and feel as if God is reaching out to me and kindly taking me by the hand into his garden. Some of the more prominent things I discover about myself are:

1. I have learned to play by the rules of manhood from older men in my life. Such "rules" were actually never spoken. Instead I learned through observation and inference. The rules I live by are:
   - Don't feel anything.
   - Never talk about what I really think
   - Never ask for help
   - Control is my friend
   - Do it alone - it worked for John Wayne.
   - Approach everything logically and rationally
   - No mercy – either myself or others
   - Every other man is my competitor – for

Irrational Medicine

food, money, women, promotions, etc.
- Don't trust other men, especially with anything personal

With this list of criteria is it any wonder that I am challenged to create successful and fulfilling relationships?

2. I have a special talent for stuffing feelings and emotions such as fear, sadness, grief, and even joy. I can pretend that I don't feel normal human emotions and routinely use the defenses of repression, isolation, and intellectualization. Power, women, possessions, money, and success have taken the place of any authentic emotional life. I am only comfortable with feelings such as anger, and never do I speak of any feelings in the company of other men.

3. I use my intellect as a defense mechanism, but hidden behind that is the soul of a small boy.

4. When I was a child, I was constantly watching the mood in my home, and if there was trouble brewing, I would go to the basement and play or hide so I wouldn't be in the middle of it. I discover that throughout my adult life I continue to hide in the "basement" of my emotions away from other people and conflict.

5. The skills I learned in danger require the presence of danger to be effective. Since my greatest skill is getting myself out of trouble then I am at my best when I have some trouble to get out of. In a strange way I feel safer in fear and danger than I do in tranquility because I know how to survive danger. I basically have no idea how to manage peace.

Irrational Medicine

6. I fear abandonment and rejection. I worry that what I have inside may not be enough, may not measure up to the task of living. I fear my gifts, my intuition, even that my spirit is somehow tragically deficient.
7. I doubt my right to belong and grab almost anything – a job, a sexual partner, a lifestyle – and make that my place of belonging. In my desperation I lose my serenity. But no other human being can provide that belonging for me. Neither my ex-wives nor my parents are in charge of granting me a place here on this earth; my place is already given. My challenge, my work, is to honor my place in this moment, to breathe deeply in the unconditional gift of home.

As I discover these things about myself my mind begins to be intrigued with questions that I have long since put aside because I did not believe I had a right to ask them. Questions such as "Why am I here?" and "Who is God?"

New Beliefs and Values

Eventually I come to the realization that my life is a journey in which I find my way by assuming responsibility for my behavior. This is self-determination. When I lapse into psychological or learned helplessness and stop taking charge of my life, I become a victim of my emotional reactions. Refusing to be guided by guilt, shame, and anxiety is a major step toward making room within myself for reason and love. The weekend has provided me with the following tools to do this:

Integrity: I create for myself a true, grounded

Irrational Medicine

sense of integrity. I am who I say and I am. I do what I say, and I say what I do. My words and actions are congruent. I keep my agreements and promises with others. When I can't keep a given agreement, I renegotiate a new agreement before the old one expires. My integrity is never in question.

Accountability: I am willing to account for and be responsible for the choices I make in my life and the consequences or impact of those choices. I stop making excuses. I stop blaming others. I give up my need to be a victim. I finally understand that I create my reality and my life. I stop blaming others for what I've created or failed to create in my life.

Telling the Truth: I create a practice of telling myself and others the truth. Period. I get out of the denial, delusion, and fantasy that I use to manipulate reality, and I get into the truth. I practice telling myself the truth about myself and my choices. I no longer accept half truths, partial truths, lies, deceit, manipulation, or coercion from myself or others. I understand that my truth is not THE truth; it is my truth. So I practice compassion in telling my truth to others. I don't have to explain or defend my truth to others. I simply have to know and live what is my truth.

Emotional Literacy: I allow myself to feel and experience the full expression of my emotions: joy, sadness, fear, anger, and dozens of others. I use my feelings, as well as my brain, to help me make decisions. I express my feelings appropriately. I practice compassion and gratitude daily.

Mission and Purpose: I develop for myself a

Irrational Medicine

clear vision of the kind of world I would like to see and create a mission statement for myself that speaks to what I am willing to do each day to bring that kind of a world into being. I live my mission truthfully and passionately, and I stop waiting for others to take care of or fix what is important to me. It is up to me to create the kind of family, relationship, community, government, country, or world I would most like to be a part of.

Watching the progression of men doing their work and especially through my own experiences, it seems as if months or even years of psychotherapy are condensed into a single weekend. Each man, as he makes a connection with his past, is able to process his dysfunctional issues. Our memories lose their power to set off inappropriate emotions. When one person does his work, it inspires others to do the same. One man after another steps up to face his demons. After watching so many men do their work, it occurs to me that healing is contagious.

When it is my turn, I take a journey that investigates the lingering scars and wounds of my childhood that continue to color my emotional landscape. I learn to speak the truth about my sorrows and hurts and to describe the inner geography of my heart with clarity and precision. I feel a surging readiness to be healed. The scars of childhood that have cast long shadows deep in my heart are released. I make the following pronouncements:

    I claim my right to walk upon the earth.
    I claim my right to say "No" to those things I do not want.

Irrational Medicine

I claim my right to live my life according to my own wishes.
I claim my right to speak up for myself.
I claim my right to live the way I see fit.
I claim my right to make choices.
I claim my right to be happy
I claim my right to eliminate those things from my life that do not make me happy.
I claim my right to speak and live my truth;
The truth of who I am, why I am here, and how I choose to live.

When I finish my session an elder staff member comes to me and says: "Bless you for what you have gone through, here is something to help you remember your journey." He hands me a small rock from the camp grounds that symbolizes mother earth. I take that rock and hold on to it like it is a piece of gold.

Sunday Afternoon

Can you imagine entering Heaven and then being asked to leave? That's what it is like for me on Sunday afternoon as the weekend comes to a close. I feel like I am where I belong, and I do not want to leave. Some kind of knowledge has been made available to me. It is as if some circuitry in my brain and my heart has been hooked up to a deep, deep memory bank of love and peacefulness. I feel so close to the 27 other men that have gone through the training with me that I do not want to leave them. As I leave the camp I know without a doubt that something has shifted inside of me. I know for the first time in my life that I am no longer a little boy in a man's body, but truly a man in a man's body.

Irrational Medicine

I know that I have just been through the most powerful experience of my life and that something this powerful was necessary in order for me to overcome my childhood conditioning. I have learned to trust and love men, something I have never done before. For the first time, I am able to drop my mask of competence and sophistication in front of other men.

I have also discovered that I have available to me a wealth of healing practices bequeathed from the spiritual traditions of the world. I have found in my bones the male mode of feeling and have learned to speak in male voice, trust male intuition, and love men nonsexually. It feels like a homecoming and has strengthened my true self.

I cry for the first five hours of the trip back to Columbus because I feel as if I have been yanked from the arms of God.

Back To The Real World

January 30, 2002: As I return to the real world after the New Warrior weekend things seem to change. I attend my ex-mother-in-law's funeral, and find myself going up to people and initiating conversations. I am actually able to join in with groups of people without be self-conscious. At work I initiate conversations with coworkers and they look at me like they aren't sure who I am. My staff members are very tentative every time they ask me for something, like I am someone they are dealing with for the first time. My oldest son John and I go out to eat and people keep staring at me throughout dinner. I actually find myself wanting to interact with other people. Boy is this strange for me. I definitely feel different, changed inside.

Irrational Medicine

My best friend Cedric Marsden sees the difference immediately and signs up to attend the next training which is being held in Idaho. Within several weeks some of my other friends Glen Sterling, Michael Figg and John Neuhart sign up for the training based upon the changes they see in me.

I-Group

As each day passes I practice what I learned on the weekend, and as I refuse to empower self-destructive feelings they wither within me. I know if I pamper them, it's like throwing steak to a dog; they grow in their demands and their boldness. My goal is to continually supplant guilt, shame, and anxiety with rationally chosen ethics, reason, and love.

One of the tools a New Warrior has is a weekly meeting with fellow Warriors called an Integration Group (I-Group for short). Men meet each week to exchange joys and sorrows and all the other emotions we have experienced during the week. It's purpose is to help each man integrate the training on an ongoing basis and to help each man deal with any issues that may be coming up for them.

A typical Monday evening meeting begins with men gathering outside by 6:00 p.m. to form a circle where a ceremony is conducted to build the sacred container for the evening. Back inside, we sit in a circle as we listen to each man speak his truth. We speak with statements that use "I", to reflect our responsibility for our opinions and judgments; we speak of our feelings, and avoid intellectualizations; we promise confidentiality to all who attend, so that each may speak freely, openly, and honestly. Any man may pass on any process, or decline any question or request, or may leave at any time, without hindrance

Irrational Medicine

or interference. No man is ever intentionally shamed or rejected or abandoned emotionally, for anything that he expresses. Each man feels safe to own and express his emotional self.

Occasionally, a man may get in touch with anger, or sadness, or fear, and will express this with energy and vigor; sometimes a man will cry, or yell, or laugh out loud, or shout, or beat on the floor, or just sit in silence. Sometimes, a man may request a specific process, such as a role-playing interaction, or a symbolic gesture, or a guided visualization, in order to break through an emotional block or sustain an emotional state until a resolution can be reached or an emotional charge can be discharged. This goes on until 8:30 p.m., when we gather together into one circle again, express where we are at now, bless and thank each other for the evening, and depart.

There are some healing elements at play in I-Groups. They allow men to express their thoughts and feelings without being judged (acceptance). They help men become aware of themselves, of their feelings, and of why they behave the way they do. Men in the group become aware of unhealthy ways they may be relating as well as their thinking process and which patterns are unhealthy. From other's sharing, the members also learn healthy ways of thinking, relating and behaving. I-Groups teach members how to listen. Men also continue to learn to accept and understand their feelings of hurt, anger, hate, sadness, and frustration as well as feelings of happiness, joy, and peace. The group helps men develop skills to express these intense feelings in healthy, acceptable ways.

February 9, 2002: I have my first Reiki session with Tere since going through my Warrior training. Without saying what it is, I ask her to hold my stone from the camp. When she takes it in her hands she

Irrational Medicine

flinches and begins to cry. She says, "This holds the energy of many warriors; it possesses the power of each charka, and it comes from a sacred place." I then tell her about the New Warrior Training Adventure and my weekend.

When she starts the session and touches my face I can feel a tremendous heat. She says, "Are your teeth hurting you?" I say, "Yes ever since I returned from the weekend." She says, "Past life memories are stored there. During your meditation ask that the pain be taken from you but that the lessons remain."

As the session continues she sees a tribe of Indians sometime in the 1700s, a time prior to the white man running the country. She says that I am a powerful leader and that I am second in charge of the entire tribe. She sees that I have tremendous wisdom and it comes through as a bright yellow light as bright as the sun. I am in love with a woman and wish that she would love me as much in return. She dies of a snake bite and I went on a killing rampage and abused my power. But I had to go through this in order to grow. I make amends, settle down, and share my wisdom with my tribe. I live a long time and became an Elder and am given my own territory to control. But I never love another woman.

She feels a very strong energy in my left arm. My right arm is very tight and she gets the message that "I need to be flexible to eat." Afterwards she comments about how different her visions were. Usually it's like she is an observer looking in. She says that with me it seems like she is in the scenes and actually living them.

Tere says the healing energy in my body is very strong and asks if I can go with her next Saturday to do a Reiki session on a woman who has a brain tumor.

Irrational Medicine

    I have no idea what I am suppose to do or how to behave but I go with Tere to help her with the session. Her client is in the last stages of brain cancer and is so feeble that she can not leave her house. Tere conducts the session telling me when and where to place my hands. When I place my hands near the ladies head they begin to shake violently. I can not control them in any way. It feels as if I am holding a live electrical wire and I can't let go. It scares me because I have no control over what is happening. I am glad when the session is over because I know I have just experienced something well beyond me and I want to get out of there as soon as possible.

    March 5, 2002: During my session with Dr. Fleetwood I express concern that I may never be able to have an unconditional loving and intimate relationship. Dr. Fleetwood says, "Relationships happen on many different levels. You should look for a woman with whom you resonate and have some attraction to. In the past you have only had the "attraction" to your partners. You fell in love with Linda because she had the happy attitude, bright, open personality that you wanted. A truly loving relationship cannot be based upon attachment or neediness. If it is, both parties get lost. You are capable of such a relationship because you have had 20 years of emotional growth in the last 3 months. You must approach any relationship as a self contained person, one that would be just as happy living alone. Each person should be as concerned with the mission and growth of the other as they are of their own mission and growth. They are together because they want to be together not because of some role to play or need to satisfy. If you love as a Warrior you will not have a problem loving unconditionally."

Irrational Medicine

Later in the day I have a session with Tere. She works on my root chakra because the remnants of my fundamentalist religious background are still there keeping me impoverished and meek. She says, "That's not the way it is anymore. Meditate with the intention that you can have, do or be whatever you want." Tere says after the session, "Internally you are in a state of schizophrenia. You are changing so much so fast that you don't even know who you are."

Chapter 8

Awareness Of An Enemy

A monk was asked, "What do you do there in the monastery?" He replied, "We fall and get up, we fall and get up, we fall and get up."
- St. Benedict

For the next few months I do well as I continue to integrate the lessons from the New Warrior Training Adventure weekend. But the side effects of the drugs begin to really wear on me. I walk around in a fog, a confusing mixture of anxiety and sedation, a kind of agitated fatigue and depression. As my condition continues to deteriorate the doctor blames it on my "mental illness" rather than on the mounting adverse drug effects.

Reading is suddenly beyond my grasp. I usually read three or four books at a time and now it is impossible. I read the same passage over and over again only to realize that I have no memory at all for what I just read. I can no longer keep track of where I am in each book.

Eventually I ask myself "Why don't I feel better?" It doesn't matter how many years go by, how much therapy I participate in or how much I try to achieve that elusive thing known as enlightenment, that happy place where all the talk is of lessons learned and inner peace, as each day passes I am feeling worse and worse. When I first started taking antidepressants I was euphoric; now life is such a struggle. Although I want them to be different, my

Irrational Medicine

thoughts are self-defeating. Though I like to proclaim myself as a positive person, I constantly criticize myself for even minor things. I feel utterly helpless, overwhelmed by feelings of helplessness. I've had years of therapy, and psychotropic drugs, and I still feel troubled and that my life is beyond my control.

    I wait and wait for the return of good moods and enthusiasm, but except for rare appearances, all I can manage is anger, despair, and bleak emotional withdrawal. At times I am immobilized by depression, unable to get out of bed, and profoundly pessimistic about every aspect of my life and future. Despite my tremendous personal transformation I continue to endure a confusing mixture of anxiety and sedation, a kind of agitated fatigue or depression. My condition deteriorates and my psychiatrist blames it on my mental illness.

    May 2002: Because Ritalin is a controlled substance my doctor is not allowed to write a prescription with several refills attached. Instead I have to visit him every thirty days in order to get a new Ritalin prescription. During my monthly visit I complain that my mind has turned on me: it no longer finds anything interesting or enjoyable or worthwhile; it is incapable of concentrated thought and turns time and again to the subject of death. Dr. Allen responds by increasing my dosage of Ritalin from one to two timed released capsules in the morning. My doctor tends to live by the adage: "When in doubt, medicate."

Ritalin Effects and Abuse

    I have slipped into a chronic abuse pattern with the Ritalin because I need it to keep going and to avoid the inevitable crash. I can't get to sleep at night then need the drug to get going again in the morning.

Irrational Medicine

Ritalin really appeals to me because I am so busy. When I take the pills my mind sharpens, and I have energy to go about my day.

July 2002: I complain to Dr. Allen: "I have noticed a pattern each day of taking the medicine in the morning and feeling euphoric, having more energy and endurance and mental sharpness through the afternoon. Then around 4:00 p.m., I start to experience heightened fatigue, poor concentration, irritability, and depression. My mood crashes, and my mind grinds to a halt. I lose all interest in my work, friends, or anything else. It is all I can do to make it home and plop down in front of the television, where I usually sleep for at least two hours. Then I get my second wind and stay up until midnight." Dr. Allen says, "You must not be getting enough Ritalin. So I'll increase your dosage from two to three pills each day."

(Later I discover that this scenario is commonly referred to as interdose withdrawal. The time released Ritalin, which I take once a day, leaves my system around 4:00 p.m., leaving me exhausted. I also discover that Ritalin can make people psychotic and depressed, producing a zombie like inhibition of feeling and spontaneity. The American Psychiatric Association describes Ritalin dependence as causing irritability, attentional disturbances, and memory problems, as well as a variety of more severe psychological disorders, including depression and social withdrawal. With larger doses, the agitation tends to become more frequent and more obvious. Certain antidepressants used in combination with the stimulants worsens agitation. Ritalin can profoundly disrupt the reticular activating system in the core of the brain, causing impairments in energy level, alertness, and responsiveness, causing a person to be

Irrational Medicine

apathetic and less aware of the world around them. Constant exposure to Ritalin can produce tolerance, or a reduction of the drug effect. Thus, the drug loses its tendency to produce euphoria, requiring increased doses to achieve an equivalent effect.)

The longer I take Ritalin the more I suffer from anxiety, loss of impulse control, and impaired judgment. I can't walk into a store without buying something, anything. My initial feelings of euphoria give way to severe, suicidal depression.

At home I stop answering the telephone and take endless hot baths and naps in the hope that I might somehow escape from the deadness and the dreariness. I become suspicious and distrustful. I also develop a motor tic under my right eye. As I use more and more Ritalin I experience a reduction in spontaneous behavior and a flattening of my emotions. I respond less, exhibit little or no initiative and spontaneity, offer little indication of either interest or aversion, show virtually no curiosity, surprise, or pleasure, and seem devoid of humor. In short, I am relatively but unmistakably humorless, and apathetic. I am sad, tearful, depressed, and simply tired all of the time. I go through cycles of feeling energized and exhausted. I have difficulty sleeping. My doctor fails to recognize these adverse drug effects and mistakenly believes my depression has returned, thus increasing my antidepressants, which further worsens my mental condition.

What Life Is Like

The hallmark of my life is a persistent sad or empty mood, sometimes experienced as tension or anxiety. Life lacks pleasure. I go through the motions of eating, work, and play, but the activities seem

Irrational Medicine

hollow. Eventually I withdraw from these activities, feeling too tired and tense to participate. There is a constant nagging fatigue that is always with me. In most cases I feel unable to focus and am unproductive at work.

I go through long periods where I eat too much, alienate everyone close to me, and am barely able to go to work. I wake up each morning hating the thought of facing the day and my life. There are many times I think of suicide, but I can't forget John Bender's words so many years ago about the impact it would have on my children. For many long periods life seems so miserable, hopeless, and joyless that I wish for a way out. While committing suicide is not an option, getting hit by a bus or some other natural disaster is appealing. A low grade, fitful instability has become an integral part of my life. The only relief I get is my Reiki sessions, my time with Dr. Fleetwood or when I sit in my I-Group meetings.

August 2002: During my monthly 30 minute visit with Dr. Allen I say, "I have noticed several times that after walking up the stairs at my house I am out of breath. Sometimes I have to lie down. I also can't sleep at night and I am starting to experience nightmares, sweating, and abnormal jerking movements of my body." Dr. Allen says, "You might want to get a heart work up."

(Later I discover that combining antidepressants and Ritalin can suppress central nervous system function, thereby impairing respiration, and can cause cardiac arrhythmias, leading to heart failure.)

The hardest part of each day is simply getting out of bed in the morning. If I can do that much, I have a fighting chance of getting through the day. Before long I am hopelessly out of control. I cannot

Irrational Medicine

follow the path of my own thoughts. Sentences fly around in my head and fragment into phrases and then only individual words remain. My mind races from subject to subject, but instead of being filled with the exuberant and cosmic thoughts, it is drenched in awful sound and images of decay and dying. During these agitated periods I become exceedingly restless, angry, and irritable. It never occurs to me that I am suffering from drug side effects.

    I feel defective, as if my brain is not working right. I have a sense of something gumming up the mental works. This feeling makes me even more susceptible to my psychiatrist's pronouncements about chemical imbalances in my brain and further encourages my reliance on him. Through it all I deny my lack of interest in life and personal problems. I declare "I'm fine, never been better," but I am no longer thinking straight. I no longer go into my back yard and work in the garden or even cut the grass. Instead I spend all my free time in front of the television hiding from life.

Things Go Bad At Work

    Work has been stressful at times, but it has always been challenging and stimulating rather than overwhelming. But my professional life starts to fall apart because of my unexplainable sadness and overwhelming fatigue. I cut down on my overtime at work and sleep in on the weekends, but my weariness becomes more debilitating. I am finding it impossible to concentrate and I am losing control of my emotions. I go to work and pretend to be well when I am not and go through the motions of being pleasant when I feel dreadful. Mental exhaustion has taken a

Irrational Medicine

long terrible toll on my mind, body and spirit. I manage people for a living but I can't even manage myself. I am having a crisis in my emotional responses and all my doctor can do is add or increase my medicine.

On most days as soon as I arrive at my office, I shut the door and avoid the company of coworkers. I cancel numerous appointments on the pretext that I am too busy. As time goes on, my behavior becomes increasingly strange. The meetings that I cannot avoid make me extremely ill at ease. I feel incompetent and exposed. I find everybody else better informed, more creative, more dynamic than I am. I know it is only a matter of time before my inadequacies will be revealed. Once alone back in my office, I shut the door and cry, all the while telling myself that it is ridiculous to get so worked up. I expect to be dismissed from one day to the next and wonder what I am going to say to my family.

To make matters worse I get a new boss who tries to make a name for himself. He is a temperamental, unpredictable person, and there is no altering the situation. I learn to avoid him by learning his habits, confining myself to written communications, working with my door closed, and keeping a low profile at meetings. When I am forced to be with him, he is just insufferable. Eventually he gets tired of my tactics and starts dealing directly with my subordinates to get things done. I don't have the mental clarity or energy to fight back and confront him so I sit in my office with my door shut. My new boss becomes angry at my poor productivity and threatens to demote me to another job – or fire me altogether. Over the past year I have gone from being productive and successful to being a despondent wreck in danger of losing my job.

Irrational Medicine

Life Is A Struggle

Some mornings in the shower, where I try to organize my day, thoughts are so fast that I can't remember the beginning of a sentence halfway through. Fragments of ideas, images, sentences, race around in my mind like squirrels in a cage. Finally, they become meaningless thoughts that I cannot recognize. I want desperately to slow my thinking down but cannot. I feel infinitely worse, more dangerously depressed, despite all of the medicine. I do not recognize my mind and certainly cannot trust it. My self esteem is very low, I feel like a helpless victim of fate.

Life is a struggle that is not worth fighting, not merely for my own sake. I fail to find meaning beyond the weariness of being myself. I can find no reason other than my children and mere survival to go on living. I am exhausted to the depths of my being and no longer wish to go on. I pray for a gentle, painless, peaceful death. Suicidal thoughts and impulses are constantly present like a form of lust. Somehow I manage to get through my work and family duties, but my mind is never free of pain, a pain that has but one solution – self extinction.

I don't want to kill myself, but I don't want to live either. I just want out of this mess. An old friend of mine named Doug Morrisey was a scuba instructor before he died of brain cancer three years ago. Before he passed on he told me about a way of committing suicide that would be painless and quite pleasant. He referred to it as nitrogen narcosis. He said you put extra weight on your belt, go to the deepest part of the ocean and just sink to the bottom with the oxygen turned completely up. As you drift further down in the

Irrational Medicine

water your blood stream fills with nitrogen. As you drift deeper and deeper you begin to hallucinate and experience a state of euphoria then you pass out and just die. The promise that on the other side of depression lies such a beautiful death continues to intrigue me.

Electroshock is an Option

September 2002: At this point if I don't have the Ritalin I can't function during the day. As soon as I get out of bed in the morning I take all my medicine. It is my energy source.

After several months of higher antidepressant and Ritalin dosages I complain that my mood isn't any better. Dr. Allen says, "A lot of patients who have been severely depressed for many years actually get worse the longer they are on the drugs. It seems to be the natural course of depression. If this trend continues with you we might want to consider electroshock therapy – that is if things don't begin to turn around soon." I say, "I thought electroshock therapy was abolished in the dark ages." He says, "Oh no, while the use of electroshock therapy has declined it is still being used in extreme cases."

I consider his words for a moment but something about them scare me.

October 2002: Once again I voice my concerns to Dr. Allen. I say things like the medicine isn't working, I don't feel the energy and euphoria that I once did. He says a bunch of reassuring things, explains over and over again how carefully he is working with me to get the right combination – he admits that psychopharmacology is more an art than science and it takes time. This time he adds the antidepressant Effexor to my other medicine.

Irrational Medicine

November 2002: I complain about agitation, anxiety and trouble sleeping. I feel overwhelmed, have lost ambition and hope, feel alone and alienated, am tormented by guilt and thoughts of suicide. In general life stinks, and there's nothing I can do about it. So Dr. Allen prescribes the tranquilizing drug Buspar again.

What's Going On?

December 2002: I attend the New Warrior Leadership-1 training in Indianapolis Indiana. My roommate is a chiropractor from Cincinnati, Ohio by the name of Jack Armstrong. He questions me about all the pill bottles in the bathroom. After I explain what each one is for he says, "Man, someday you might want to try to get off the medicine but be careful because after so many years your body has grown accustomed to having the drugs and will rebel when you try to stop." I say, "It would be nice to get off them. Each month I spend $643 for the pills and it costs me another $120 for a doctor visit. But my doctor says that my depression is a disease and that I will need the drugs for the rest of my life."

Coming Off The Medicine

During the middle of December I realize that I am running out of my medicine. I call Dr. Allen's office but get an answering machine telling me that the office is closed until after January 3, 2003 because the doctor is on vacation. So I count out my pills and figure that if I only take half of my usual daily dose of each medicine I can make it last until January 3.

Irrational Medicine

After two days on reduced dosages of the medicine I begin to have more energy and my mood improves. For the last half of December I am feeling better than I have in a long time.

January 3, 2003: When I see Dr. Allen to get new prescriptions for my medicine I explain to him what happened and how I cut back on the dosage of all the medicine. I ask why did I feel so much better on less medicine. He snaps at me, "You never should have cut back on your medicine like that. It was just a fluke that you felt better with less medicine. I want you to take these new prescriptions, fill them and get right back on your usual dose of medicine!" Then there is a shutdown of his concentration as he writes my new prescriptions. My little voice inside says "Something isn't right, this guy is only interested in pushing drugs. I need to get a second opinion."

January 27, 2003: I make the 72 mile drive to Dayton to visit my dad at his home. When I walk into the family room I am shocked to find an old, wore out man sitting on the couch. At first glance I do not believe this is my dad. He looks so sick and has aged so quickly. He looks just like my grandfather. He says it is just the flu and refuses to go to the doctor.

A Second Opinion

February 2003: A friend of mine recommends a new psychiatrist named Dr. Richardson. It is very hard to get an appointment because he only sees a handful of adult patients and for some reason is phasing them out. He wants to specialize in treating children with ADD. But as a favor to my friend he agrees to accept me as a patient.

During the 45 minute session I express my concerns that the drugs are having a dulling effect on

Irrational Medicine

my mind, suppressing my vitality, and producing lethargy in me. After some more questions Dr. Richardson proclaims that I am not depressed but that I have Bipolar Disorder.

He explains that Bipolar Disorder is an illness marked by extreme changes in mood, thought, energy and behavior. It is also known as manic depression because a person's mood can alternate between the mania, which are the highs, and depression, which are the lows. These mood swings can last for hours, days weeks or months and can range from extreme energy to deep despair. Referring to the DSM he references the following symptoms:

> Manic symptoms include: Severe changes in mood-either extremely irritable or overly silly and elated. Overly-inflated self-esteem; grandiosity. Increased physical and mental activity and energy. Decreased need for sleep-ability to go with very little or no sleep for days without tiring. Increased talking-talks too much, too fast; changes topics too quickly; cannot be interrupted. Distractibility-attention moves constantly from one thing to the next Hypersexuality-increased sexual thoughts, feelings, or behaviors; use of explicit sexual language. Increased goal-directed activity or physical agitation. Disregard of risk-excessive involvement in risky behaviors or activities
> Depressive symptoms include: Persistent sad or irritable mood. Loss of interest in activities once enjoyed - social withdrawal. Significant change in appetite or body weight. Difficulty sleeping or oversleeping. Physical agitation or slowing. Loss of energy. Irritability, anger, worry, agitation, anxiety. Feelings of worthlessness or inappropriate guilt. Difficulty

Irrational Medicine

concentrating – indecisiveness. Recurrent thoughts of death or suicide. Unexplained aches and pains.

He tells me how to stop taking the Wellbutrin, Depakote, and Buspar and then instructs me on taking a new medicine called Lamictal. He plans to continue my Ritalin at the current dosage level.

(Later I find out that mania or bipolar disorder is the most extreme manifestation of antidepressant induced stimulation. In other words, my bipolar disorder is drug induced.)

After leaving the doctors office I start to think there really is no cure for my condition, that happiness will be a never ending battle for me and one I will have to fight for as long as I live. I wonder if it's worth it. I can survive almost anything, as long as I see the end in sight. But this affliction is so insidious, and it's impossible to ever see the end.

Landmark Forum

February 2003: I attend the Landmark Forum in Columbus. It is a different experience for me because it is not experiential like the other trainings I have been to. It is more of a guided dialogue between the course leader and the attendees. It is three days long and is conducted in a casual environment. The class has about 125 people in it and I see a lot of people aggressively engage the material, participate and produce remarkable results in a short period of time.

I learn that while I think of myself as open-minded and objective, in fact my view of the world is filtered and even obscured by pre-existing notions and ideas. These ideas are directly connected to my upbringing, values, and past experiences. These filters

Irrational Medicine

profoundly color my relationships with people, circumstances, and even myself.

I learn about the human tendency to make up stories about what happens to us. Over time the story I tell myself becomes the way it is – the reality I know. These stories can limit what is possible in my life, robbing me of much of my joy and effectiveness. When I can separate what happens from my story or interpretation, I discover that much of what I consider to be fact may not be that at all. Situations that were challenging or difficult become fluid and open to change. I find myself no longer limited by a finite set of options, and able to achieve what I want with new ease and enjoyment.

I discover that I relentlessly judge myself for who I should be and never accept myself just as I am. Whatever I am feeling in this moment is judged against some mythical ideal of how I "should" be feeling, what I "should" be doing, and who I "should" be. If I feel hurt, I think I should have been healed by now; if I feel frightened, I think I should be stronger; if I feel sad, I think I should be happier. Every moment every breath of my life is subtly judged as unacceptable. Measured by the standards of who I should have been by now, I constantly fall short. The judging mind insists that I become other than who I am, and I fall victim to the violence of that requirement.

I learn about Rackets, an unproductive way of being or acting that includes a complaint that something shouldn't be the way it is. While my complaints may seem justified there is a certain payoff – some advantage or benefit I receive that reinforces the cycle of behavior. At the same time, there is a steep cost too.

Basically the training explores a new view of

Irrational Medicine

language that alters the very nature of what is possible. Language is seen as a creative act. Listening and speaking take on new dimensions and unexpected power. They are the instruments of creation.

The Landmark Forum helps me frame my life in a new way and leaves me with an ability to relate to life with new freedom and power. The Landmark Forum is really about a moment-by-moment approach to being alive.

Chapter 9

Your Instincts Have Gold In Them

The visible world is the invisible organization of energy.
- Physicist Heinz Pagels

At this point in my life I feel almost no joy in life, I have no hope, no ambition, I feel stuck, powerless, and perennially sad – and worst of all I think this is the normal way to feel. I have experienced a global deterioration of my mind and mental faculties but I have no idea that it is caused by the very drugs that I credit with keeping me alive.

March 2003: After he has a six week long bout with the flu, we finally convince my dad to see his family doctor who immediately sends him to Good Samaritan Hospital in Dayton. After a full week of tests the results are that he has three blocked coronary arteries, an aortic aneurysm and a gallbladder that needs to be removed. The diagnosis is given to the family as if it is no big deal. Dr. Liim the surgeon says: "We'll do the heart first then we'll work on the aortic aneurysm, then eventually the gallbladder after he gains some strength." My father consents to the treatment plan but since he is only 65 years old all of these problems at once seem overwhelming, especially to a man who has never been in the hospital before.

Irrational Medicine

March 24, 2003: After the heart surgery Dr. Liim comes to the waiting room and says, "It went well. I did five bypasses and clamped an aneurysm on the backside of the heart, but he still has a leaky valve. He also has an irregular heartbeat but that is common after bypass surgery. But now I am concerned about the possibility of the aortic aneurysm starting to grow because the heart is pumping stronger."

After the surgeon leaves the waiting room I begin to wonder why did he do five bypasses instead of the three in his original diagnosis and how could he have missed the aneurysm on the back of the heart and he never mentioned a leaky valve. Also why didn't he tell us about the possibility of the aortic aneurysm growing after the surgery? The surgeon had to have known it was a possibility when he first mentioned the surgery to us.

(I would later see this process of gradual disclosure over and over again in my dad's treatment. Doctors would tell us enough to get our cooperation or to satisfy our curiosity but it would never be the complete story.)

New Discoveries

After the heart surgery something goes terribly wrong. The first day Dad is in intensive care he comes in and out of awareness and seems to recognize the family. Then he just sleeps all of the time, and we begin to ask why. At first we are told it is the anesthetic, but after several days this excuse wears thin. Eventually a neurologist is called in to examine him. The doctor mentions in passing that one in a million patients suffer a stroke after such a surgery,

Irrational Medicine

but he doesn't think it is the case with my dad. He orders some tests to verify what is happening.

Meanwhile I am scheduled to attend the Landmark Advance Course seminar for four days in Cincinnati. Since Dad is out of surgery and there is nothing I can do, I decide to go ahead and attend the class. The timing is perfect because during this four day training I discover two amazing things about myself that make an immediate difference in my life.

The first thing I learn is that I have a program playing in my mind that I must do as I am told. When I was six years old and my mother was hospitalized my dad took me to my cousin's house and sat me down in the sandbox. I chose to sit there and not run after him as I made up the story that I should do as I am told. Through the years I have had trouble dealing with authority figures. Rather than speaking my mind I simply do as I am told to do. This keeps me in the box in more ways than one.

The other epiphany is that during that same incident I made up the story in my little head that he did not love me. Based on those events I constructed the story that I was a bad boy for what I had done to my mother and that my dad did not want me around. Since I was only four years old, I didn't understand that he needed to return to work. I missed the fact that my father was experiencing a tremendous sense of loneliness and sadness himself because his wife was in the hospital and he was left with two young children to take care of. At the time my father was only 26 years old and he had a job that he couldn't afford to lose. That had to be a lot of responsibility for someone so young.

So based on this story I spent the rest of my life looking for evidence to prove that I am right. It is a natural human tendency for the mind to prove it is

Irrational Medicine

right. Looking back, this story has tarnished my relations with, and the way I felt about, my father for over 40 years. Because of it I built a wall between us.

Once I realize what I have done I begin to remember some of the good things about my childhood. I had blocked out memories of events like the two of us going fishing, or when he would go camping with me while I was a Boy Scout, when he helped me in the Pine Derby and how he participated in the Indian Guides.

My father is not a bad man, but I have been only looking for the evidence that proves he is. How many times do "our stories" impact our lives? Stories about what things people's actions mean. Stories that may have no basis in reality yet we live our lives as if they are completely true and accurate. I now realize that the stories we make up about what happens to us impact our lives in dramatic fashion. So I need to be damn sure that the stories empower me rather than destroy me.

When the training is over I return to the hospital and find that my dad has been moved into a private room. This time I look at my father as a totally different man.

Pat, my step mother, tells me that the doctors have determined that he had a stroke during the heart surgery. I remember that one-in-a-million comment and wonder if the neurologist knew what happened and he was just setting us up for the bad news. Was this gradual disclosure again?

Over the next few days I read "get well" cards and letters sent to my dad from friends and coworkers, and I begin to realize how respected and loved he is by people I don't even know. A picture of a kind and considerate man emerges before me. Because I have released the story that my dad does

Irrational Medicine

not love me, I am able to see who he really is for the first time.

When I start to know him as a human being, I begin to see that no one is all bad, and I start to be more compassionate to myself as well. In a curious way, this is the start of courage. I realize a lot about myself through this experience.

Not Getting Better

Dad is sleeping all of the time and just isn't waking up. Days pass, and we are hoping to talk with the specialists on his case. But the neurologist doesn't return our pages and never comes by. There are several doctors on his case but none of them come to see us and explain what is happening. We have no clue what is going on.

Each day I go to the hospital to check his progress, and each day he seems to be worse. His breathing is very labored, and he does not know who anyone is. When I ask what is happening, the nurses say it is the effect of the stroke, and it will take a while for us to see any progress.

April 3, 2003: I am sitting by my dad's bed when the surgeon comes in to make his rounds. He yells my dad's name as he shakes him trying to get him to come to, but gets no response. I ask him what is going on. He says, "Don't worry your father has been given a sedative and is just sleeping." Right then the head nurse walks in. She says, "Mr. Wilson has not been given a sedative." Dr. Liim argues, "You are wrong he is sleeping all the time because of the medicine." She counters back, "I have been taking care of Mr. Wilson and I know for a fact that he has not been given any sedative."

I am shocked, amazed, and somewhat

Irrational Medicine

entertained that such an argument is taking place right in front of me. Eventually they both agreed to check the chart but neither of them returns to the room. Instinctively I know that the head nurse is right. She spends a lot more time with my father than the surgeon does.

Later that day, while making my 75 mile drive back to Columbus, I replay the scenario over in my head. I wonder what kind of egotistical maniac can stand in front of a patient's family and argue with the head nurse to try and prove he is right. He is willing to ignore the facts or not consider another opinion just so he can be right. He isn't concerned about my father as much as he is concerned about being right.

When I get home, I call my step-mother and tell her what I think about the care my dad is receiving. I am not convinced that he is in the best of hands at Good Samaritan Hospital. She agrees with me and expresses her frustration at not getting any response from his doctors. She then asks if I would take over my dad's care and work with the doctors on her behalf. I agree and say the first thing we need to do is move him to another hospital where the doctors might actually come and see him or at least talk with the family.

What Have I Done?

When I hang up the phone I begin to wonder how on earth can I do such a thing. Doctors are like Gods. They know what is right and what is wrong. What justification do I have to question their authority? But deep down I know that if I don't do something my father isn't going to get better. I know that he is slowly dying and that something needs to be done. I am also angry at the doctors for ignoring us and not telling us what is going on.

I am very worried that I will go to the hospital, start voicing my concerns and then cave in to the doctors telling me that everything is all right and that I just need to be patient. Deep down I know that isn't an option and there has to be more that can be done. I call Tere and we talk for a while about my situation. She encourages me to stand up for myself and for my dad.

As soon as I hang up the phone I sit down at my computer and type out an action plan using the principles I have learned from all of my personal growth training. I promise to carry this with me and refer to it whenever I begin to doubt myself and what I need to do.

The actual sheet I used:
TRANSFORMATION PLANNING SHEET : Save My Dad's Life

Priority: I must accomplish this	**Date:** April 3, 2003
WHAT isn't good enough...	**WHY isn't this good enough...**
My dad is lying in a hospital and is not getting any better. The doctors are not working as a team to heal him and they are not respecting me or my family by keeping us informed of his prognosis.	He may never be the man he once was or he may even die from malpractice.
What I am pretending...	**What I am HIDING...**
That the doctors know what they are doing. That I don't have a say in the matter because they are in charge. That the surgeon is competent and the neurologist gives a damn.	I am frightened that my dad will not survive this. Or if he does he will be no more than a vegetable. I am afraid to speak up because then I will not be doing as I am told.
The IMPACT this is having on myself and others...	
I am a nervous wreck because I don't want to lose my father. He is too young to be in a nursing home. It is devastating my grandmother and stepmother. It is preventing dad from a living a life he loves.	
My Probable Almost Certain Future	
My father will die in the hospital.	

Irrational Medicine

The POSSIBILITY that I am inventing for myself and my life is the possibility of...	
My father getting the best treatment available and making miraculous progress toward recovery and walking out of the hospital.	
The REASON (feeling) I want this possibility is...	
I want to demonstrate how much I love my father by taking a stand for his health and full recovery.	
The REASON I want this result is...	
I want to get complete with him through an enrollment conversation.	
My new BELIEFS about this possibility are...	
It is my right and duty to get the best possible care for my father and I can only do that by getting their attention. It is my right to stand up for who I am and what I want. My father will get only the treatment that we will tolerate. I am going to have to say things that may upset people, but it is my duty as a loving son because it is my father's life I am fighting for.	
My New Future (Measurable results)	
My dad walks out of the hospital feeling like a new man with more energy, vitality and hope for a bright future. He is able to return to the police force and retire like he had planned.	

Massive Action Plan

Objective	Get my dad appropriate medical care so he can recover completely from his surgery and stroke.
Task	Consult with Dr. Botti: What information do I need to be 100% clear about before I make a decision?
Objective	Solicit help from Hospital. "We are not satisfied with the care my father is receiving. I need to know what is going on."
Task	Who is in charge at Good Sam and can help me with my father's care. Contact Customer Service/Consumer Relations.
Obstacle	**Doctors are not informing us what is happening.**
Task	Identify all doctors on his case, their areas of expertise and their diagnoses.
Task	Obtain phone numbers for each doctor.
Task	Contact each doctor to discuss the case. What is it they know and what are they doing to help my dad.
Obstacle	**Suspect that doctors are not treating him properly or as a team.**
Task	Request a group consultation with all involved.

Irrational Medicine

Obstacle	**Doubt the competence of the surgeon** Argument with head nurse over sedation. Why hadn't he checked his chart prior to seeing him. Statement about blood clot will always be there. There's nothing that can be done about it.
Task	Ascertain the competence of Dr. Liim and the credibility of his statements.
Task	What type of surgeon is Dr. Liim?
Obstacle	**Doubt the competence of the neurologist** Observations: Did not call Pat even after numerous messages left to do so and was paged by the hospital staff. Has not consulted with the family.
Task	Determine why we have been ignored.
Outcome	**Option #1:** By 3:00 PM arrangements made to move dad to Miami Valley and replace every doctor on his case.
	Option #2: By 4:00 PM arrangements made to move dad to Riverside Hospital in Columbus and replace every doctor on his case.
	Option #3: Replace non cooperative doctors by 2:00 PM and have a status report of his condition and a solid treatment plan approved by the family.
	Option #4: Meet all doctors consulting on his case before 12:00 PM April 4, 2003 with a status report of his condition and a solid treatment plan approved by the family. I want a double positive prognosis or I will find someone else to help him.
Task	Obtain assistance from attorney to observe dad's treatment so far.
This or something better now manifests for me in totally satisfying and harmonious ways for the highest good of all concerned. Thank you God.	**To be Completed: April 4, 2003**

The Battle Begins

April 4, 2003: At 8:00 a.m. I walk into the hospital and ask to speak to a customer service representative about my dad's case. I am told that I need to talk with the lead doctor on his case, that all modifications to care have to be coordinated through him. In this case it is his family physician Dr. Lang. After several forceful phone calls by 10:00 a.m. I am

Irrational Medicine

sitting across from doctor Lang in a conference room.

I proceed to tell Dr. Lang that our family is not happy because we have not seen any of the other doctors on my dad's case, we don't know what is going on with his condition and that we want to transfer my dad to another hospital. He says: "I understand your concerns but moving your dad is not a good idea in his condition, and the doctors involved have been working diligently on his case." I begin to doubt that what I am asking is reasonable, and I quickly review my document, then restate my case and insist that he make the arrangements, but he refuses. Then as my grip on my plan tightens something wells up inside of me and I say: "Dr. Lang, I respect your opinion but if you refuse to do as I ask, I will fire you and find someone else who will do what I am asking." When he sees how serious I am he relents and agrees to handle the arrangements. At that moment something shifts in me because I have stood up to the closest thing to God on this planet and won.

By 4:00 p.m. my dad is transferred to the Critical Care Unit at Miami Valley Hospital on the other side of Dayton where he is greeted by a critical care specialist, a neurologist and several nurses to get him settled in. They run numerous blood tests and discover that he has a low grade infection in his lungs, which is why he is sleeping so much. They immediately start treatment and within 24 hours he is awake and recognizes us for the first time in several days. Then the neurologist Dr. Black runs tests and tells us the stroke is not that bad and she suspects that most of his problems have been from a lack of oxygen due to the pulmonary infection.

After a few days of good progress, and relatively good news from his doctors we are starting to see

Irrational Medicine

hope and can envision an end to this nightmare. Then his cardiologist, Dr. Brewster, comes in, and I ask when my dad can return to work. He just looks at me and says quite calmly: "Your dad has congestive heart failure and will never be able to return to work." This is the first time any doctor mentions that his heart is that bad. We were led to believe that it isn't that serious. Once again we are hit with gradual disclosure. Dr. Brewster says "We will wait 12 months before surgery on the aneurysm, 6 months at the earliest. Basically, your father is retired now. His heart is so bad that he will never be able to return to work."

Another Teacher Shows Up

By now the ordeal with my dad has taken quite a toll on me. Making the 150 mile round trip to Dayton on a regular basis has worn me out. The constant worry about his condition as well as the stress from dealing with doctors and nurses, who seem to have other things on their minds, have drained me. The relationship with my boss is very strained. A couple of times he suggests that I take a leave of absence because of all the time I am missing from work. I also notice that I hold my breath. Tere warns me that this is the way I suppress feeling the emotions in my body.

During a Saturday morning breakfast with old friends Glen Sterling tells me about a massage therapist he has been seeing by the name of Char Young. He says, "She is a body-centered therapist who has developed a unique integrative healing approach that combines bodywork, breath and emotional dialogue. She has deep insights and skills to unravel the stories that we hold deep within

Irrational Medicine

our bodies and how they effect our emotions and life as a whole. She has an ability to work with trapped energy in the body." That little voice inside of me says that this woman is someone I need to see. So later that day, I call her and make an appointment for Thursday.

For the first 30 minutes Char and I just talk to get to know each other. "I want to work with you because I am hurting; despite a lot of medications, I am anxious, depressed, confused, frustrated, and just plain unhappy about my life. My biggest complaint is that I suffer from exhaustion. My ultimate hope is to improve my life and find some good feelings – maybe even some joy."

Char says, "Most of the people that come to me are afraid to feel the depths of their sadness. They are afraid of their suppressed rage and of their suppressed panic or terror. It is my job to help you confront these unknown terrors and learn that they are not as threatening as they seem. We experience emotions in our body, not in our head. Chronic tension is the physical equivalent of fear. Every chronically tense muscle in the body is a frightened muscle, or it would not hold so tenaciously against the flow of feeling and life. It is also an angry muscle, since anger is the natural reaction to forced restraint and the denial of freedom. Suppressing feeling is a deadening process that diminishes the body's vitality. Suppressing one feeling suppresses all others. If you suppress your fear you suppress your anger. Suppressing anger results in the suppression of love. People who come to me, regardless of how successful they may be, have had their spirit broken to the degree that joy is an alien feeling. Their body movement is extremely limited due to severe muscular tensions binding them like chains."

Irrational Medicine

To become an effective guide Char has undergone such treatment herself which resulted in self-realization. She explains our work together will be a journey of self-discovery. She warns me: "It will not be quick, or easy or without fear. The life of the individual is the life of his body. Since the body includes the mind, the spirit and the soul, to live the life of the body fully is to be mindful, spiritual, and soulful."

When I lay down on Char's table, she feels my heart and says "It's a good thing you have come to see me. The tension is so high in your body that you are probably close to having a heart attack." Because of what I am going through with my dad and the pressure at work, this statement does not surprise me at all. As she massages me she says: "Right now you are suffering from considerable tension in your chest, lower back, legs, which bind and restrict you, destroying your ability to express yourself fully. Feelings are energy, and they can be bound by chronic muscular tension. A person who doesn't breath deeply reduces the life of his body. If he doesn't move freely, he restricts the life of his body.

The session with Char is very similar to a normal deep tissue massage, except a little more painful. But I feel better afterwards. I am more energized; my body moves a little more freely, my mind is a little clearer. This lasts a few days and then like a rubber band that is stretched and then released I return to my uptight self.

The Story Continues

April 14, 2003: My dad continues to make great progress and is moved to the rehabilitation floor of the hospital, under the care of Dr. Wats, to deal

Irrational Medicine

with the residual effects of the stroke. They work with him every day getting him up and walking, but then on the 20th he becomes restless, experiences a lot of pain and his urine is very dark. Pat and I notice right away that something is wrong because his condition deteriorates rapidly. We question Dr. Wats and he orders tests the next day.

April 24, 2003: Dad is very restless and in extreme pain, but there are no test results yet. A Gastro-Intestinal doctor comes in later that afternoon and does an impromptu bladder ultrasound and says that the pain is caused by a full bladder so they put in a catheter.

April 25, 2003: At 8:00 a.m., five days after we noticed a change in dad's condition, the doctor says that he is suffering from a bladder infection. At 2:00 p.m. they finally start him on an antibiotic for the infection.

April 26, 2003: We are told he also has a bacterial infection and has passed a blood clot.

April 27, 2003: His doctors inform us he has Vancomycin-Resistant Enterococcus (VRE) and needs to be isolated. In order to visit him we have to wear yellow gowns, plastic gloves, and blue masks. Dad does not know who we are anymore, and he just babbles when he talks.

Finally Pat and I have had enough, so I contact patient relations and demand that Dr. Brewster and Dr. Shawl be called in for consultation and that he be moved back to the Critical Care unit. I explain that his condition has deteriorated rapidly since being moved into the rehab unit and that I don't feel as if he is getting appropriate care from the doctor assigned to his case.

In the Critical Care unit, they determine he has another infection in his lungs in addition to the

Irrational Medicine

bladder infection. After a few days of treatment my dad is coherent and talking again.

Something Else Goes Wrong

May 1, 2003: Dr. Shawl, the critical care doctor, tells us that the aortic aneurysm is now 7.8 cm, growing and in danger of rupturing. He says that surgery is not an option because my dad's heart is not strong enough to withstand the operation. One option is to place a stint in the area with the aneurysm and hope that it will slow down the expansion.

A few days later I am walking down the hall of the hospital and come upon Dr. Shawl on the telephone talking to another specialist. Since it is in the hallway of the hospital I figure I have a right to stand behind him. I overhear him say, "His wife is reasonable and will probably go along with the treatment but he has a son that is unreasonable." When he hangs up the phone and turns around to see me standing there Dr. Shawl looks as if he has just seen a ghost. I say, "We need to talk."

I get Pat and we meet the doctor in a conference room. I ask Dr. Shawl, "What will happen to my dad?" He answers in general terms. I press him to be blunt and tell me if my dad didn't have the aneurysm what would be his chance for survival from his heart condition. He says, "Your dad has less than a 25% chance of surviving more than a year with his heart condition." Then I say, "If he only had the aneurysm to deal with what would be his chances?" He says, "Your dad has less than a 25% chance of surviving from the aneurysm." I say, "So basically my dad is not going to make it." His response, "That's probably true." I thank him for his feedback and tell him we will get back with him tomorrow.

Irrational Medicine

That night I make the 75 mile drive back to Columbus and sit down in my living room to think. As I sit there in complete silence I begin to feel a profound objection to physicians who deliver death sentences. I feel a certainty that what happens to us is much more in our own hands than we might suppose. I decide that the doctor is wrong, that my dad is going to live and that I will find a way.

I go to my office, get on the internet, and start researching aortic aneurysms. I find that the Cleveland Clinic, which is 2 hours north of Columbus, is the number one hospital in the world in the treatment of aortic aneurysms. They also specialize in secondary treatment, which means that they correct the mistakes of other hospitals.

May 5, 2003: I call the Cleveland Clinic and talk with a nurse in the Vascular Center. Later that morning, I drive back to Dayton and meet my stepmother for lunch at the hospital where I tell her about my research. I say, "If Dad has any chance at all, it is at the Cleveland Clinic." She agrees, so we sit down with Dr. Shawl and I explain what my research has turned up. I tell him that we want to move Dad to Cleveland. Dr. Shawl says, "I am familiar with their program and I believe it is a good choice on your part."

At first his comments don't register with me then I recognize a major issue. If he knew about the Cleveland Clinic why didn't he suggest it in the first place? Why didn't he say there were other options for treatment? If we had gone along unquestioningly with his recommended treatment, Dad would not have been given the option of the Cleveland Clinic. I thought it was a doctor's job to provide the best treatment possible and give a patient all his options?

I drive back to Columbus that afternoon, and

Irrational Medicine

by 4:00 p.m. I get a call from the hospital telling me that my dad has left for the airport where a medical transport jet is waiting to fly him to Cleveland.

A New Beginning

May 6, 2003: I leave Columbus at 4:30 a.m. and arrive at my dad's hospital room at the Cleveland Clinic at 7:00 a.m. His first day there is remarkable. I count 13 doctors that come in and examine him. Everyone from neurologists to coronary specialists and physical therapists interview him to understand his case. While this is going on Pat is in Dayton at Miami Valley Hospital collecting records, x-rays and test results. The transfer happened so fast that they had sent nothing with him.

After several days the vascular surgeon determines that an operation is the only option because the aneurysm is larger at the bottom than at the top. I ask him about typical treatment options, and he explains that they prefer to use stints and only in extreme cases do the surgery. I find that interesting because the doctors in Dayton first proposed surgery and only suggested using a stint when surgery was not an option: totally different approaches. I also find out that Cleveland has a procedure where they can do both the open heart surgery and the aneurysm surgery at the same time.

I ask how can they recommend surgery on him right now because his doctors in Dayton said that he would never survive it. The vascular surgeon says, "We do these types of surgeries all of the time and our experience says it can be done." So we agree to have the surgery.

May 17, 2003: We are visiting with my dad and still waiting to hear when the surgery will be

Irrational Medicine

scheduled. I notice a loaded syringe laying on his bedside table and wonder why it is there. He is having a great day, he is awake, talking coherently and in a good mood. He isn't agitated and is content watching television. It's one of the few days since he's been in the hospital that he can actually carry on a conversation. Later that morning Pat and I decide to get some lunch in the cafeteria. When we come back we are shocked to find him knocked out. He isn't just sleepy, he is drugged. By now we can recognize the signs.

    I notice that the syringe on his bedside table is gone. I ask the nurse what happened, and she tells us that there is a standing order for Haldol (a sedative) to be used if my father is agitated. I explain that we had been with him less than an hour ago and that he showed absolutely no agitation and was in good spirits all morning. The nurse said it was orders. I make it clear to the nurse that I believe he is drugged just so she wouldn't have to deal with him. She does not respond.

    I am mad because I have been cheated out of quality time with my dad. He sleeps all afternoon and well into the evening. Consequently his sleep cycle is interrupted causing him to be up all night, which makes him agitated the next day.

    Most of the time when he is awake he is with us in body, but his soul is in some way lost. The deeper feelings and tenderness are gone. He is like another person. I suspect that the Haldol makes him less emotionally spontaneous and passionate. He is more shallow and relatively inert, or blunted. This blunting makes him less troublesome to the nurses and a better patient to the doctors - it is restraint by chemical means.

    Later I find out that Haldol is a tranquilizer and

Irrational Medicine

falls into a group of drugs called antipsychotic or antischizophrenic or neuroleptic. Neuroleptics are the most frequently prescribed drugs in mental hospitals and are widely used in nursing homes, institutions for people with mental retardation, prisons, and in tranquilizer darts for subduing wild animals. When Dad was on Haldol he displayed apathy, disinterest, and followed the medical staff's instructions without question.

May 19, 2003: At 10:00 p.m. we are finally told that the surgery will be 12:20 p.m. the next day.

May 20, 2003: Pat and I arrive at my dad's room the next morning at 7:00 a.m. as usual only to discover that he has already been taken to the surgery prep area. They changed the schedule, but no one had bothered to let us know. We hustle down to the surgery waiting area, hoping that we might get to speak to him, but it is too late. They have already started the preparation process.

The surgery begins at 9:15 a.m. and is suppose to last six hours, but at 11:45 a.m. we get a call from the doctor in the surgery waiting area. Since it has only been a little over two hours it shocks us, and we think something has gone wrong. The doctor says, "We did not want him under anesthesia any longer than necessary so we had a team of vascular surgeons working on him at the same time. We cut out the section with the aortic aneurysm and replaced it with a synthetic Dacron graft. Just continue to wait for a few minutes while they transfer him to the Surgical Intensive Care Unit (SICU), then you can see him."

We waited and waited until finally at 3:00 p.m. I ask the surgery desk about my dad's status. They check their computer system but are not able to locate him. They make several phone calls and finally

Irrational Medicine

locate him in the SICU. When we check in at the SICU, we are told he has been there since 12:00 p.m. So we were in the surgery waiting area for 3 hours waiting and worrying about his condition needlessly.

May 25, 2003: After a few days in intensive care unit, my dad is transferred to a room in the Vascular Unit of the hospital. We request a sitter be placed in his room like there was in the Heart Unit. We are told that before a sitter can be assigned, a manager has to approve it. We are also told that they are short staffed and really don't have anyone to spare. We are assured, though, that he will be assigned a sitter the next night. After being notified that he has fallen out of bed May 27th and May 28th, we ask if the sitter had been present. We were informed that a sitter had never been assigned to him.

May 29, 2003: I get a call at 3:00 a.m. telling me that my dad has fallen out of bed again. I get in my car and make the 2 ½ hour drive to the hospital. After talking with Pat we decide it's time to get him back to Dayton for the rest of his recovery, so someone from the family can be with him all the time. Later in the morning I meet with his case worker and tell her that I want my dad transferred to either Miami Valley Hospital or Kettering Medical Center in Dayton. I specifically and unequivocally state that he is not to be moved to a nursing home and that Miami Valley or Kettering are the only acceptable options.

Arrangements are made by the case worker for his transfer to Kettering via ambulance. When the ambulance arrives their manifest lists Auburn Hills in Kettering as the destination. When I question the destination, I am told that they do not know why Auburn Hills is listed but that the location is indeed Kettering Medical Center. Later that evening I drive to Dayton to the address given by the case worker and

Irrational Medicine

discover that it is Auburn Hills nursing home in Kettering - no affiliation what so ever with Kettering Medical Center. I am shocked that he has been transferred to the wrong facility totally against the wishes of the family.

The next day we have him transferred to a different nursing home in Dayton that has a rehabilitation facility on site.

The Hara

I have been seeing Char at least once a week, sometimes twice a week, as time allows. Each session lasts between one and two hours. At times she touches certain muscles and terrible feelings flood my body. I just want to get up off the table and run away, but I wait out the pain and things get better. Each session leaves me feeling a little more alive, a little more free, a little more energized. But she has to keep reminding me to breathe. It frustrates me because I can't breathe the way she insists I should. It's as if something is stuck in my abdomen that keeps me from breathing that deeply.

As Char begins to work on my body, she observes: "Your body is so tight, and your breathing is very shallow. When a person loses the pleasure of being alive, his breathing is restricted and his interest in life declines." That certainly explains a lot of what's going on in my life right now. She goes on, "The surrender to your body involves nothing more than allowing its full and free respiration to occur. The fear of surrender is connected to holding the breath. When you limit the amount of oxygen the body absorbs, it reduces metabolic activity, decreases energy and diminishes feeling. When there is a place for breath in the body, there is a place for belonging for our spirit.

Irrational Medicine

We may begin to feel our belonging in the breath – here we may take sanctuary, here we begin to feel our place in creation. Taking refuge in each breath of our life, in each beat of our heart, we find a quiet place of belonging. This refuge, this sanctuary, is neither given nor taken away by the chaotic demands of an unpredictable world (in other words, peace). This place belongs to us, and we to it. It is where we make our home. You have lost touch with God because you have lost touch with the God within you – you get in touch through the breath, the Hara. You need to get feeling into the belly so you can sense your guts and into your legs so you can sense them as mobile roots – it is called grounding. A grounded person feels he has the solid support of the earth under him and the courage to stand up or move about on it as he wishes. To be grounded is to be in touch with reality."

As Char forces me to work on my breathing, I suddenly become nauseated and start coughing uncontrollably. At first I resist the idea of coughing and throwing up, but Char points out that this is my body's way of not holding in and getting it out. The experience shakes me, and I am surprised to find that coughing so violently immediately calms my anxieties. Char says: "If the body is allowed to come alive, it will find its own way to release its tensions."

Back In Dayton

In the nursing home/rehabilitation facility, days turn into weeks. My dad heals from the surgery, but I cannot see any significant mental progress. Each day I go to see him he just lies there not demonstrating any typical human functions such as love, concern for others, empathy, creativity, initiative, autonomy, rationality, abstract reasoning, judgment,

Irrational Medicine

planning, foresight, willpower, determination, or concentration. He expresses no emotion and cannot take care of himself.

Then one day Pat questions his doctor as to why my dad is still on the tranquilizer Haldol. When he cannot give her a good reason she insists that the drug be stopped. Within days my dad is able to walk, talk, dress, and feed himself. I walk in to visit him and am shocked at the progress he has made seemingly overnight. It is obvious that the drug Haldol had physically and neurologically blotted out most of his ability to think and act as well as his personality. Now he is able to actively participate in his rehabilitation and begins to make tremendous progress.

Since his doctor cannot explain why the drug is necessary by the diagnosis in his chart, I suspect it is merely used as a chemical straightjacket - a means of pacifying my dad to keep him manageable. I wonder how many months or even years we would have visited him hoping for some improvement without realizing that it is a drug keeping him from healing.

It's interesting to note that my dad does not remember any of the time from his first surgery up until the tranquilizer Haldol is stopped at the nursing home. He cannot recall any of the hospitals or doctors during the time he had been given the tranquilizer.

Going Home

July 11, 2003: After four months, three hospitals, two rehab facilities, and so many doctors I lost count, my dad goes home.

I am quite relieved seeing my dad at home for the first time in months. But I can't help but wonder what could have happened if we were told all the facts

Irrational Medicine

in the beginning. How things could be different if his doctors didn't play the game of gradual disclosure? Their priority seemed to be to rush him into submission of a treatment plan and turn him into a submissive patient.

If we had known all of the facts up front, we would have been a whole lot more selective about the hospital and surgeon we used. If we had been given all the facts we could have made better choices. Instead the doctors let us stay in the dark as along as possible only providing minimal information. By the end I was paranoid about gradual disclosure, about bad news dripping out. When a doctor spoke to us, it always left me wondering, "Will there be more?" The failure of doctors to impart information seemed to come partly from ignorance and partly from their attitudes toward patients. Many doctors did not seem to feel obliged to tell us everything. Instead they controlled the flow of information in order to achieve certain ends, such as encouraging the acceptance of treatment.

There was also a real difference in the level of care and attention from one hospital to another, from one doctor to another. It seemed the longer we were at a hospital or worked with a specific doctor the greater the decline in attention and care.

I am convinced that if we had been willing to accept their prognosis at Good Samaritan or Miami Valley hospitals eventually they would have turned around and said "Nothing more we can do for you. Go home and wait to die." The practice of gradual disclosure by the doctors cost us time, money and could have cost my dad his life.

Final Thoughts

Irrational Medicine

Throughout this ordeal I begin to see that doctors are not the infallible creatures that I have always believed them to be. I begin to question everything they do, and when I get an answer I don't like, I get a second and sometimes third opinion. I also start to question the way certain drugs are used and how they are given without much consideration as to the impact on the patient, just the end result the doctors want.

My beliefs about the medical profession in general begin to change. I realize that there is an incredible amount that doctors just do not know. As well as a lot of information they withhold from patients intentionally. The standard mode of operation seems to be 1) keep the patient calm, 2) do not tell them much, 3) use compassion and a tranquillizer.

I learn to question doctors and treat them as hired help. It's our responsibility for our own health, and doctors are there to help but it's ultimately our own decisions as to how to proceed with treatment. Doctors may think they're doing the right thing, but that's not necessarily the case.

Now I begin to wonder what my own doctor is not telling me. Is my psychiatrist purposely withholding information about the dangers of my drugs for fear that I will refuse to take them? Does he believe that I need the medication so bad that he prescribes it without providing sufficient information for me to make an independent decision?

Chapter 10

Can I Have My Golden Ball Back?

The dissenter is every human being at those moments of his life when he resigns momentarily from the herd and thinks for himself.
- Archibald MacLeish

    My work with Char continues. She reminds me often that I am my body. Since the body includes the mind, the spirit and the soul, to live the life of the body fully is to be mindful, spiritual and soulful. Her therapy does not attempt to help me adjust to anything. Rather, it helps me overcome the effect of turmoil by restoring my body to its natural state of relaxation. In the process of her massage therapy I reexperience the deprivations and pains of my childhood and youth. To these I react with rage, sorrow and sometimes laughter. I am able to protest the inequities of my life by kicking and screaming.

    My body is bound by so many tensions that there is little spontaneous movement and, therefore, little feeling of any kind. The massive tensions in my body are a formidable obstacle to feeling and require intensive physical work. Char frequently comments on how hard I make her work. She will push a certain muscle and I cry, scream out in pain, or cough uncontrollably. She presses a different muscle and I break out in uncontrollable laughter.

Irrational Medicine

During my next session with Char she explains the connection between the body and mind: "The chronic tension in your muscles is connected to unresolved emotional conflicts stemming from childhood. These conflicts operate in the present as long as the tensions persist in the body. The chronic tension is like a prison that prevents the free expression of your spirit. As a child you lived in fear and deadened yourself to not feel the pain or the fear. Deadening the body eliminates the pain and the fear but you imprison those impulses in your body." I am surprised by her comments because I have never mentioned any kind of childhood abuse or trauma. She then presses hard into my back and I scream as if I have been stabbed with a dull knife.

Char says: "Go ahead and yell, 'Leave me alone!'" In a moment I am possessed by feeling. My kicking becomes stronger, my yelling louder when suddenly I break down crying. When the crying subsides, I turn to Char and ask: "How did you know that was what I wanted to say?" She answers: "I just had an intuitive sense. We all have suffered losses and hurts that our minds may accept but our bodies do not. The body cannot release its pain except through a violent catharsis."

The Will

During another session Char focuses on my back. She says, "For survivors, like you, surrender to the body is strongly resisted because it brings up the most painful and frightening feelings. You probably learned that you must not express emotional pain and did what every other survivor learns to do – dissociate from the body and withdraw into the head. Cut off from the body, you don't feel vulnerable. By

Irrational Medicine

identifying the self with the ego, one also gains the illusion of power. Since the will is the instrument of the ego, one truly believes where there is a will, there's a way. Or one can do whatever one wills. This is true as long as the body has the energy to support the ego's directive. But all the willpower in the world is no help to a person who lacks the energy to implement the will."

I have had back pain for as long as I can remember but I never dreamed it was the result of stored energy. I have spent most of my life operating through my will and it is tiring.

Char helps me notice the tension in my body by selectively applying pressure on tense muscles to produce an immediate release. She says, "Under a steady pressure a contracted muscle will often let go. The tension becomes unbearable and the muscle relaxes." Then she digs her elbow into my shoulder muscle and I feel an unbearable pain. I scream: then I begin to cry. Both of these releases have a positive effect on my mood.

Physical Changes

As the repression is lifted and the suppression of feeling eases through Char's work, my body slowly comes fully alive. I can see physical changes in my body such as better definition of the muscles she works on during each session. Each session leaves me feeling a little more energized and a little more comfortable in my own skin. Each session makes me stronger and more open to life, more able to surrender to my body. Each session I breathe a little deeper.

I am more in touch with my body than I have ever been: more aware of its tensions and more conscious of its weaknesses. By the same token, I can

Irrational Medicine

sense my feelings more easily. Through my work with Char I make contact with more sadness and anger than I have ever experienced. The release of these feelings has an exhilarating effect. There are times when my heart opens up and I feel radiant and glowing. More significantly though is the sense of well-being that I often have. My body gradually becomes more relaxed and stronger.

    I keep working with both Tere and Char because they seem to help me with different aspects of myself. I feel good for a little while after my sessions with them. Then when I start to feel bad again I go in for another session. But there is also a glass ceiling on my mood. It seems that no matter how much work I do I can not feel joy, like something is holding me back.

Time To Change

    I am experiencing problems with my judgment, insight and abstract reasoning. My mood and feelings are unstable. I can't concentrate: it's hard to pay attention to conversations, to focus on reading anything complicated or to work consistently on a project. I find it difficult to remember things such as a list of items to get at the grocery, the time my children said they were coming home, or the name of the person who just left a phone message. I find it difficult to do simple operations on my computer, to find the word or phrase I want, or to remember the name of some familiar object. At times it is hard for me to find my way around the main building at work even though I have been all over the building before. I find it hard to follow complicated questions or directions, to think about more than one thing at a time, or to carry out a logical sequence of thought.

Irrational Medicine

While I used to think of myself as "quick" I now seem "slow." I become baffled by conversations involving more than one person. I am less able to handle everyday stresses such as getting my children ready for school, trying to arrive at work on time, being late for an appointment, falling behind in a project or being interrupted. Later I will learn that these are classic signs of drug induced psychoses.

I find myself getting unusually annoyed, frustrated, or irritable, and sometimes hurt people's feelings without meaning to. I also find myself becoming unexpectedly angry or aggressive. I spend money I don't have and screw up my bills. (These drug-induced problems are called paradoxical reactions or disinhibition.)

I also have trouble falling asleep and staying asleep. I do not wake up refreshed. I don't care about anyone or anything as much as I used to; my feelings often seem blunted; my internal landscape is bland and less colorful; I feel indifferent, apathetic, and lethargic. I don't have the same amount of mental or physical energy that I once did and I get tired and discouraged much more easily. I am sluggish and lethargic and exhausted by the evening. I feel not just fatigued but "ill," "worn out" "blah" – as if I have the flu or some other debilitating physical ailment all the time.

I have lost any enjoyment of life and only have feelings of gloom and hopelessness. I feel as if I have lost my spark when it comes to thinking about solutions to problems, new ways of looking at things, or even what to do with my time on a free Saturday afternoon. Too often I feel bored.

I have trouble figuring out how I am feeling and why I am feeling that way. Friends and family members comment that I am not looking well, or

Irrational Medicine

inquire whether I'm feeling ill, when I haven't even noticed anything wrong. My feelings seem to go up and down without any reason, and I have more trouble controlling what I feel and when and how I show it. My most frequent feelings are of agitation, anxiety and panic.

    I begin to suspect that the "miracle drugs" are not curing me and that years of taking antidepressants and Ritalin have cost me some of my mental sharpness, especially my ability to focus and concentrate. I cannot stand the pain any longer, I am fed up with the bone-weary and tiresome person I have become - one would put an animal to death for far less suffering. I am just beginning to understand that not only my mind but also my life is at stake.

    July 15, 2003: Thanks to my experience with my dad I am now a more questioning patient when I meet with Dr. Richardson to get new prescriptions. I ask the doctor if he can be sure of the bipolar disorder diagnosis. I question him about my condition, the drugs he recommends and their side effects but he is a careful man weighing what he says and will not volunteer information. He refers to the DSM and espouses the theory of biochemical imbalance. But when I ask how he can prove that I have a biochemical imbalance he admits that it is only medical theory. There is no blood test, or CAT scan or any other test that can be run to prove that I have a biochemical imbalance or even that the drugs fix such an irregularity. There is no marker for depression. The individual's personal feelings remain the basis for diagnosing depression, or bipolar disorder. They think antidepressants work on the biochemical because some people respond positively to the drugs. I ask about stopping my medicine. He says that will never be possible and reminds me that I

Irrational Medicine

have tried it in the past and failed each time.

I reluctantly take my prescription refills from the doctor because I need the Ritalin to survive, but I vow to find a way to be free from these "miracle drugs."

Homeopathy

July 17, 2003: Since traditional medicine does not seem to be working I decide to seek the assistance of a homeopathic physician by the name of Rosana Dominques. After graduating from medical school Dr. Dominques practiced traditional medicine for 5 years before she became dissatisfied with the system and started searching for a holistic approach to heal the sick. She went back and obtained her homeopathic credentials.

Homeopathy was once the most popular form of medicine used in this country. Into the late 1800s and the early 1900s, a large percentage of the hospitals throughout the United States were actually homeopathic hospitals. Homeopathy is based on the philosophy that the body, mind and emotions are not really separate and distinct, but are actually fully integrated. Based on this perspective, a homeopath seeks a remedy that fits all of a patient's physical and psychological symptoms. Mental and emotional symptoms are often given greater weight or meaning by homeopaths than are physical symptoms. As a result, homeopathic remedies, when correctly prescribed, can sometimes produce major healing effects in patients that involve not only a disappearance of chronic physical symptoms but also a profoundly positive shift in mental and emotional states. Homeopathic remedies can address many illnesses, especially those for which conventional

Irrational Medicine

medicines have failed. Homeopathic remedies can successfully treat psychological as well as physical problems, including anxiety, depression, and in certain cases even mania and schizophrenia.

Homeopathy is primarily a nonphysical, or energetic healing modality. The practice believes that human beings are more than just a physical body. Human beings are unique energy systems with many complex energy-control systems helping to regulate and maintain the health of the physical body. A homeopathic physician attempts to match a specific homeopathic remedy with the symptoms of the patient. Homeopathic remedies are specially prepared doses of intensified energy, prepared from pure, natural, animal, vegetable or mineral substances that are listed in the Homeopathic Pharmacopoeia. They are presented in the form of granules, tablets, pellets, or liquids and are thought to resonate with the body, triggering a positive healing response. This response gently, and effectively, heals from the inside out. Only the correct selection of a particular homeopathic remedy will produce any effect upon the patient at all. Because homeopathic remedies are so extremely dilute, there are no side effects experienced from taking an "incorrect" remedy; there is merely no effect at all.

My first session with Dr. Dominques lasts for two hours. She asks many questions about my specific problems as well as general physical, emotional, and mental makeup. She asks questions about specific symptoms, on which side of the body the symptoms tend to occur, preferences in foods and whether certain foods or beverages tend to aggravate my condition. She asks questions about my temperature and climate preferences, mental and emotional tendencies, and any history of early

Irrational Medicine

psychologically traumatic experiences. She pays special attention to unusual symptoms that most conventionally trained MDs don't quite know what to make of. For example, she really focuses on the fact that I tend to wake up every night at four in the morning with feelings of dread. Strange symptoms seem to actually have great significance in helping her focus in on a remedy that is appropriate for me. Things like craving sweets, or night sweats or the need to be by the seashore or other strange preferences or aversions seem to have deeper meaning to her.

She explains "Symptoms are the language of a disease - the body's attempt to balance itself. Homeopathy does not seek to remove or suppress symptoms. Its goal is to recognize and remove the underlying cause of these symptoms. This is why I will work toward understanding your entire being, which includes body, mind and emotional state, before prescribing a remedy. The goal of the remedy is to encourage the body to return to a natural state of balance and health. Like the missing pieces of a puzzle, homeopathic remedies fill-in the gaps in the body to stimulate a person's own healing potential and energies. When this occurs, you will have access to your body's natural strength and wisdom, so that more conventional medicines and chemical-based substances will not be needed."

I say, "I feel worse and worse every day I am on the drugs and I wonder if they aren't part of the problem. I sense that there is a cost to taking drugs, such as a dulling of my emotions, a slowing of my thinking processes, and my lackluster attitude toward life in general. My doctor merely suggests that I need larger doses or additional medications but I suspect that I need to get off them entirely. I want to be in

Irrational Medicine

control of myself rather than at the mercy of a medication. I want off the drugs so I can get my life back."

She says, "That is understandable. Psychiatric medications are first and foremost psychoactive or psychotropic drugs. They influence the way a person feels, thinks and acts. Like cocaine and heroin, they change the emotional response capacity of the brain. If used to solve emotional problems they end up shoving those problems under the rug of drug intoxication while creating additional drug induced problems."

I say, "In the past I have tried to come off the drugs, and the depression comes right back." She replies, "I suspect that your past failures at stopping psychiatric drugs had more to do with their withdrawal and rebound effects than with your own emotional or psychiatric problems. It is not going to be easy, the larger the doses and the longer the exposure to the drugs the more difficulty you can expect during withdrawal. And you've been on these things for 23 years. Letting go of a drug is bound to create physical and psychological reactions as your body begins to adjust to the absence of the drugs. After the drug is reduced in dosage or stopped, it takes time for the brain to recover. Withdrawal effects will show up during the recovery period. They are caused in part by the delay in the brain's return to normal functioning. Don't be surprised if you experience dizziness or loss of balance, nausea, vomiting, other gastrointestinal problems, flu like symptoms of fatigue, muscle aches and chills, abnormal feelings such as tingling, burning or electric shock feeling, sleep problems such as insomnia and nightmares, possibly aggressive and impulsive behavior, anxiety or agitation, irritability and

Irrational Medicine

dramatic crying spells, depressed mood and depersonalization, slowed thinking, confusion and memory problems, distressing feelings in your head, including electrical shocks, as well as abnormal sounds in your ears." I sarcastically reply: "Is that all? "No! Stopping the antidepressants and Ritalin can lead to depression and even suicidal feelings. At the same time, the knowledge that you are giving up a drug and the physical changes you are undergoing will stir up various emotions and thoughts. The drug effects may have estranged you from some of your most powerful emotions, including your sense of outrage, injustice, and self-preservation. Some of these emotions may resurface when you withdraw. Also your original problems may begin to resurface if their psychological or situational roots have been neglected." I say, "I have done a lot of personal growth work on issues in my life. Getting off the drugs will help me see how much progress I have really made." She says: "If your original problems return they will be a crucial test of your determination and abilities, as you will be challenged to accept and deal with these emotions and behaviors through means other than drugs."

  The doctor then describes the process of stopping the drugs and gives me a remedy. "Before you stop taking the drugs, it is important to lower the dose over time just as slowly as when you got on. Your brain chemistry has become used to the presence of the medication, and more than just serotonin levels are affected by this process. Other neurotransmitters, like acetylcholine, will fall out of balance. Acetylcholine plays important roles in helping to regulate actions in the stomach, bladder, blood vessels, and sweat glands. It is officially called discontinuation syndrome, which is a fancy term that

Irrational Medicine

distances antidepressants from the word withdrawal and all the terrible connotation it brings. After all, it's bad business if patients get the impression that they are addicted to their medicine and will face a difficult time if they wish to stop using it."

I leave her office with a mixed sense of excitement and apprehension. But I am willing to try anything because I have grown so tired of living like this.

The Journey Begins

July 15, 2003: I reduce the amount of my medicine daily until I completely stop it on July 14. Within twenty-four hours of my last pill I experience the worst attack of the flu in my entire life. I am overcome with vomiting and diarrhea, my body aches, my head feels as though it is caught in a vise and I have a dreadful sense of impending doom.

Despite my tiredness, I have trouble falling asleep and staying asleep. A complete physical evaluation by my family physician produces no evidence of an infection so I figure this is the beginning of the withdrawal syndrome.

I gradually recover from the flu like symptoms over the next week but I am irrational and even crazy, with high levels of anxiety. At night I have disturbing dreams that waken me in a state of panic and dread. During the day I am jittery and irritable.

On a daily basis I have to marshal every bit of willpower to regain rational control and to focus my attention on overcoming helplessness. One day I go into the office and my security badge doesn't work in the card reader. I absolutely freak out, thinking they have caught up with me, and I have been terminated. For over an hour questions race through my mind:

Irrational Medicine

how will I cope without a job, what will I do for money, how will I tell my family? Then I realize the magnetic strip on my security badge has just worn out because of the years of swiping it. I go to the security department and get a replacement badge.

A couple of days later, I am walking down the hallway at work when my body begins to feel like it is falling to the left side. I compensate for this by leaning to the right and then I feel like I am going to fall down. I make it back to my office by bracing myself against the hallway walls. I sit down in my chair and stay there for about two hours until the dizziness leaves me.

July 30, 2003: I meet with Dr. Dominques and complain about all the problems I am going through. She tries to reassure me that this is a prolonged period of re-adjustment during which the chemistry of the brain settles into a kind of new, non-depressed normal. This time she gives me a very high dose of the remedy.

July 31, 2003: Based on a recommendation from Char I decide to start seeing a clinical hypnotherapist by the name of Dr. Matt Levy, N.D.. He is a rough and straightforward 77-year-old man. I find him fascinating because he has been through the Basic seminar too and we have some common ground. One of the most incredible things about Dr. Levy is that he doesn't charge me for office visits. He says that he has been blessed and just wants to give back to the world that has given so much to him. His philosophy is that if he can help me to be happy then I can make others happy and so forth and so on.

He first tests me to see if I can be hypnotized and I can. He then asks me some questions about my symptoms. I explain, "When I am depressed I am ashamed of myself and feel humiliated that I can't

Irrational Medicine

make my depression go away. I am unmotivated and don't want to go to work or play or do anything. I feel worthless and like a failure. I am sad and feel embarrassed because I should be a better person. I feel physically weak; getting out of bed is a real chore. I also have trouble with anxiety. When the phone rings I am afraid, not knowing who might be calling, that somehow this call might lead to a confrontation I want to avoid. I am afraid to answer my door or to have people over to my house. I have trouble with relationships since I am afraid of people getting to know me. I feel ashamed of revealing my feelings and ordinarily won't talk much or allow myself to show emotion. I just pretend everything is OK, telling people what I think they want to hear, a candy coated version of the truth. I often feel sad but keep myself from crying although the feeling is always there."

Dr. Levy says, "You are the sum total of all your experiences from your birth to your present moment. If you accept reincarnation, all of the experiences of your past lives are also included. These past experiences represent all of your programming, memories wholly retained in your subconscious memory banks. Thus, your subconscious mind has made you what you are today – your talents and abilities, problems and afflictions are the result of the intuitive guidance of your subconscious. It has been directing you and it will continue to direct you, often in opposition to your conscious desires."

I ask, "Why in the opposite direction?" Dr. Levy replies, "Because the subconscious has no reasoning power. It simply operates like a computer, functioning as the result of programming. Every thought programs the computer – you have to think something before you speak or act. Thus if you are thinking more negatively than positively, you are literally creating a

Irrational Medicine

negative reality. If you are not happy with the way it is, it is time to transform your thoughts. In the future consider how much you think negatively. Start catching such thoughts and neutralizing them before they become programming data by purposely creating a positive thought about the person or situation that upset you."

He then goes through the process of placing me in a hypnotic trance. Afterwards we talk about the results of the session. He says, "I have no idea what it is but you're hiding something that you don't want to discover because you are afraid that your parents may abandon you." I say, "I can't imagine what it could be." We schedule our next session.

Chapter 11

I Look Into My Own Eyes

For whatever is hidden is meant to be disclosed, and whatever is concealed is meant to be brought out into the open.
Mark 4:22

August 1, 2003: It's Friday morning and I wake up with a terrible pain in my jaw from grinding my teeth. I get up and take an unusually hot and long shower. As I am standing there an image of an old neighbor, Katy's father, flashes through my mind and I start to cough violently. Katy and her parents lived next door to us when I was in grade school. Katy was probably 20 years older than me and mildly retarded. I liked Katy, and we use to talk across the fence in the backyard all the time. In this image Katy and I are talking when her dad walks up behind her. He is a rough old man probably in his sixties. I see him peering over her shoulder looking down at me and not saying a word. I get scared and go in the house. The coughing stops, and I finish my shower and get ready for work.

Later in my car on the way to work the image pops into my mind again. This time I cough even harder and begin to gag. I feel as if I am going to throw up. After a few minutes this subsides and the rest of my 20 minute drive to work is uneventful.

I get to my office by 8:00 a.m., shut the door and just sit there for a while reviewing my 78 email messages from the day before. At 9:00 a.m. I go to the

Irrational Medicine

break area and get a glass of water and come back to sit down in my chair. Then it hits me. I begin to cough uncontrollably. The coughs are deep, long, gagging and painful, coming from the pit of my stomach. They are like the coughs I experience when I am on Char's table during a particularly painful session. For over 30 minutes I can't stop coughing and throwing up. Then images of Katy's father and their basement flood my mind and my body starts shaking so bad I have to lay on the floor. The images are very clear: I am eight years old and alone with this man in their basement doing things no child should ever know about.

My coughing and shaking is so loud and violent that it draws the attention of other people in the office. My boss comes in to see if he can help. I tell him I don't know what's happening, but I just need some time to get my composure. Then I start coughing again. He notifies security that I need help. A guard comes to my office but I just lay there shaking. He calls for an ambulance. By now a crowd has gathered outside my office trying to maintain a balance between morbid curiosity and corporate professionalism. People offer to help, but there is nothing that can be done. I continue to shake and cough and gag.

At 10:00 a.m. the coughing subsides and the shaking slows when the paramedics arrive. They take my vital signs while asking questions about my condition. They want to take me to the hospital, but because this is happening just two days after taking a mega dose of remedy and my coughing is so similar to what happens to me on Char's table, I suspect that it is not a medical condition. I don't think a hospital will do me any good so I refuse to go. At 11:00 a.m., the paramedics decide they can't do any more for me and leave. It takes another hour before I am able to stand

Irrational Medicine

by myself. I grab my briefcase and my cell phone and head for the car.

I call Dr. Levy and explain what just happened to me. He says, "Well now we know what it is that you were hiding. All of this was caused by a repressed memory of sexual abuse when you were a child." I say, "A repressed memory? How do you know it is a real memory?" He says, "Were you in pain when you were remembering what was happening in the basement?" I say, "Of course I was: it was one of the most painful experiences of my life. My jaw pain this morning from grinding my teeth, the coughing, the shaking were all extremely painful." He says, "The pain is all an attempt by your conscious mind to divert your attention away from what is going on, to keep the memory hidden. But your subconscious mind is pushing it up to get it out in the open. Apparently the hypnosis session yesterday gave your subconscious permission to act. This is the beginning of a long road to getting you better, don't worry I will travel it with you."

I then call Char and tell her what happened and about my conversation with Dr. Levy. She says, "The way your body reacted leaves no doubt that this is a repressed memory. Remember I told you that someday you would reach a point where your body could "clear" on its own. And that's why you reacted so violently. The body remembers what the mind chooses to forget. Memories can remain stored in our bodies – in sensations, feelings and physical responses. Even if we do not know what took place, fragments of what we suffered endure. This was a cleansing of the memory from your body."

I call Tere and tell her what has happened and that I need to see her right away. At 1:00 p.m. I am on her table for a Reiki treatment. As the session

Irrational Medicine

progresses I go into a deep trance, and I see my grandfather, my brother Garry and my older brother David, who had died before I was born, standing beside the table. They tell me that everything will be all right. Then I am in the neighbors kitchen and recall the smell of their house. I am sitting across the kitchen table from Katy and can see her mother Agnes at the kitchen counter. I can tell that Agnes knows the evil that her husband does in the basement, but Katy has no idea what goes on down there. I then see my grown self in the backyard of the house on Queens Ave. in Dayton where I grew up. My adult self stands between my child self and Katy's father. I draw a Warrior's sword and tell my younger self not to be afraid because I will protect him. I then proceed to hack and slice Katy's father into small pieces and when I am done with him I use the sword to destroy his house. I tell him to never bother my younger self again. I look my younger self right in the eyes and say: "You do not have to give away your power just because someone is older or bigger or in authority over you. Stand up and fight for yourself. You are more powerful than you can ever imagine."

    I then go into my house and talk with my parents. I introduce myself as the grown up Jeff and a Warrior who has returned to give them some advice. I tell them to be careful how they treat the little me. That the child is very special, gifted, and smart. That he is being stifled by their rules and inattention. I warn them to treat him better.

    After the session, Tere and I talk about my vision. She says, "You have certainly been a survivor because of everything you have endured in your life. But now it's time to do more than merely survive, from here on you will thrive."

Irrational Medicine

Saturday: I experience a series of panic attacks throughout the day. My heart pounds and I feel sweaty, weak, faint, and then dizzy. My hands tingle, and my skin feels flushed. I have chest pain and then smothering sensations. A sense of unreality overtakes me, followed by a fear of impending doom and loss of control. I don't think I am having a heart attack but it does seem as if I am losing my mind. The attacks occur throughout the day and average 20 minutes each time. In between the attacks there is an intense and lingering anxiety about the risk of having another attack.

Sunday: I develop sores in my throat and my mouth. They are similar to the ones that I had when I was diagnosed with Chronic Fatigue Syndrome.

Monday: I call in sick to work because my lymph nodes swell up the size of golf balls. In the afternoon I meet with Dr. Fleetwood because I want to get a psychologists opinion about repressed memory. After I explain what happened on Friday she explains, "When sexual abuse happens at a very young age, the child represses all memory of the events by suppressing the feelings associated with them. Suppression involves deadening a part of the body. When the feelings come alive again, memory is awakened. The pain of the experience was so great that you left your body and lived in your head. You could function seemingly normally, but you were always in a deep state of anxiety and fear that made your life almost intolerable. Your way of survival was to withdraw emotionally while carrying on your life with almost no feeling. You existed largely in your brain. Studies have shown that male children have been sexually abused almost as much as females. The sexual abuse of a boy by an older male undermines the child's developing masculinity and makes him feel

Irrational Medicine

ashamed and humiliated. The damage to a child's personality is caused by the emotional impact of the experience. Fear, shame and humiliation are devastating feelings to a child who has no way to release and recover from the insult of this trauma. It steals their security, their trust in other people and their self-esteem. It can also set up many problems for them in later life. Many adults who were abused as children suffer from a whole range of problems. This is not because there is something 'wrong' with them. Because they have suffered a trauma, it is quite natural that this should affect them. Sometimes sexual abuse leaves adults with lasting anxiety, panic attacks, nightmares and fears. Some people suffer terrifying experiences such as 'flashbacks' (reliving some of a traumatic event). For some, sexual abuse leaves them with shame, self-hatred and depression. The betrayal of trust they suffered as a child may make it hard for them to feel safe and easy in relationships as an adult. Some people cope with the painful feelings by overuse of drink or drugs. Others may overeat or starve themselves, or hurt their own bodies to express the terrible pain and confusion they feel. Sexual abuse survivors often struggle with issues of dissociation, consent, and developing boundaries. Dissociation is a completely normal response to being hurt or feeling pain. One's mind and body attempt to get away from the hurt. Some people dissociate by "spacing out," to detach emotionally from what's going on. Dissociation helps a victim of sexual abuse survive and get through their childhood, but it often lingers into adulthood and causes problems. In most cases people find out about the abuse then try to work through the issues. But in your case you have done a tremendous amount of personal growth work and then found out about the abuse. I don't think

Irrational Medicine

that you will have much more to deal with around this issue. It just needed to come out."

Tuesday: I call into work sick because there are bumps all over my face that look like measles. It's like my body is going through every disease or affliction it has ever experienced.

Wednesday: I call into work sick because my anxiety is so high and I am coughing so much that I can barely talk. I am having incredible pain in the spot where they made an incision for a heart catheterization a few years ago. Later that day I go to see Char. She says, "Given what you have just discovered it is no wonder that you have not been able to breath deeply." Char reaches around to the back of my head and squeezes on both sides of my neck. All of a sudden I let out a series of loud and frightful screams. Almost immediately my breathing becomes deep and strong. My legs feel paralyzed so Char has me kick and scream again. All of a sudden the terror leaves me and I begin to feel tingling sensations going all through my body. Then my body gets perfectly still and I have a vision. I see my younger self and he gives me a gold ball I give him a white light. We stroll together along the water, and then I hug him, and he merges into my body. Then I morph into a beautiful brown and white mustang. Then a white light emanates from me, and I change into a solid white mighty mustang. I then run up and down the beach with incredible energy and vitality. After the session, I feel better than I have for the past six days.

Thursday: I call into work sick because I am tired, full of anxiety and I am dizzy and lightheaded.

Friday: I return to work and spend the day answering the usual "How are you doing" questions. But at night I just can't sleep. I am up from Friday

Irrational Medicine

morning at 6:00 a.m. until Sunday night at 9:00 p.m. - 63 hours without sleeping.

August 17, 2003: I have a Reiki session with Tere. Two big issues in my life are trust and balance. My root charka (fundamental beliefs about the world and myself) seems to be what's holding me back. I have always lacked the trust that no matter what happens I will be OK. Tere mentions some lingering childhood beliefs that still run me:

- I deserve to live a life of poverty and lack.
- I actually deserve to be unhappy, joyless, and always have to struggle for whatever good things may happen to come my way.
- God only loves me when I fear him, do as he commands and give up my worldly possessions.
- "Don't get too big for your britches" in other words always do what I'm told and don't think or act for myself.
- Be satisfied with what I have and don't even think about living a happier or better life.
- Don't rock the boat, just follow the status quo and stay in my place. All that's expected of me is to follow the crowd and live a plain white bread existence.
- Don't bother dreaming, an unimaginable life for me is not a possibility.

The net result is that I sabotage myself, my relationships, my finances, my job, and any other area whenever I "violate" one of these beliefs by making progress toward abundance, joy, or health. When I get rid of these limiting beliefs and let things flow to me what a wonderful life I will have. It's unimaginable what my life will be like without being held back by self limiting beliefs.

Irrational Medicine

August 19, 2003: Dr. Levy puts me under and finds that I have a split personality. He says it's fairly common in people who have been sexually abused. It's their way of coping and surviving in the world as a child. This second personality holds me back and sabotages my success because it thinks I don't deserve to be happy. I am surprised by how similar Tere's conclusions were.

Throughout this whole ordeal I make it a habit not to discuss my experiences with each healer because I do not want to influence their work or opinions in any way.

Things Start To Turn Around

The next few months I just try to survive. I see Dr. Levy every Monday, Char every Wednesday and every other week I have a Reiki session with Tere. I see Dr. Dominques once a month so she can monitor my progress. The following are highlights of some of the more important sessions.

August 20, 2003: During a meditation I come to a philosophical understanding of why I experienced physical, mental, emotional and sexual abuse as a child. I endured such atrocities to expand my skills for survival. The experiences forced me to develop a quiet strength and a resilience that has helped me throughout my life. I used this strength and power to put an end to my family's intergenerational chain of abuse. Through my determination and willingness to fight for my life I ensure that the abuse will not be perpetuated to other generations. John and Jordan my two beautiful boys are the living testimony to this daunting accomplishment.

My children, my grandchildren and my great grandchildren will not have to experience the agony of

Irrational Medicine

abuse. They are free to live with self determination, a sovereignty to be who they want to be, and a knowing of their authentic selves. My actions will have a processional effect on numerous generations so I have actually achieved the greatness which I have felt destined for my whole life. Impacting so many lives so profoundly is truly a great accomplishment.

However, I have paid a tremendous mental, emotional, physical and spiritual price to make this contribution to the world. I have been controlled by the effects of the abuse my entire adult life and have struggled for everything. I have experienced physical pain, crippling fear and anxiety, failed relationships, career setbacks and financial failures. But once again the sadness, loss and disappointments have served to make me stronger and even more powerful. My father, mother and even the neighbor who sexually abused me were all my teachers. The wives who betrayed me, the bosses who fired me, my brothers who died so young, were all my teachers.

Now as I approach my 44th birthday it is my intention to go beyond merely surviving and reach a state of self-acceptance, self-esteem and self-love. I intend to live with a satisfaction that represents the connection between my spiritual essence (soul) and my new self born of toil and struggle. I will live in congruence with my soul's aspirations representing the combined expression of my conscious, unconscious and spiritual essences. I accept and will protect my rights to self determination, to be the person I want to be, to live the life I want to live and to be treated the way I want to be treated. I deserve prosperity and to live with emotional and spiritual riches as well as material well being. I also acknowledge God's most precious gifts, my two beautiful boys.

Irrational Medicine

August 23, 2003: I get up at 5:30 a.m. and meditate for an hour. As I visualize a beautiful green field I talk with myself at age 3. I am amazed at how bright, cheerful, happy, playful and full of life I am. Then I see myself at age 5 and I tell myself "It is not your fault your mother is in the hospital. Dad only said those things because he was afraid." At age 8 I tell myself: "It is not your fault in any way that Katy's dad sexually abused you. It was all about him. You just happened to be in the wrong place at the wrong time." At age 9 I tell myself: "Despite all of these things you are still destined to have a great life and you deserve it.

August 24-25, 2003: I am so exhausted that I sleep all weekend.

August 26, 2003: This morning for about an hour I feel like there are ants crawling all over my body. In the afternoon I feel like there is an electrical current running from my head to my toes.

During another hypnotherapy session with Dr. Levy, all I remember is seeing a beautiful pond. A little later in the session I begin to cough and gag. Dr. Levy commands my conscious mind to behave and my subconscious mind to provide soothing oil to my throat to stop the coughing. After that works he brings me out of the trance. I ask Dr. Levy what had happened. He says, "Your conscious mind had completely stepped aside while I worked with your unconscious mind. But when it heard something it didn't like, your conscious mind started the coughing." He starts talking to me about the possibility of a past life affecting me. I have never believed in past lives. Dr. Levy recommends that I read the book *Many Lives, Many Masters* by Brian Weiss. He explains that it's a true story about a

Irrational Medicine

psychiatrist, his patient and past-life therapy. I pick up a copy of the book on the way home.

August 29, 2003: While leaving the office, my head starts spinning and I lose my balance. It calms down after several minutes. Then on the way home it happens again while I am driving. I manage to get the car off to the side of the road. Fortunately it subsided quicker than the first time.

September 12, 2003: I get my annual performance review today. The rating is the lowest possible - Below Expectations. I am not surprised because of all the work I have missed and the hiding I have done in my office. But I am disappointed because it means I am one step away from being put on probation.

September 16, 2003: I see Dr. Levy and he wants to do a past life regression. I read the book he recommended but I am still skeptical. He regresses me into a trance and after a few minutes I walk out of a tunnel into the coliseum at Rome. I am 35 year old Claudius Allrealis, an accountant for the coliseum. I am an orphan, single, very well off, not married and have no kids. My only companion is a Nubian house slave named Sophie. I stay home most of the time, have few friends and I am very narcissistic. One night while leaving the coliseum through a dark tunnel I am attacked by thieves. They break my back with a lead pipe. I never recover and just give up and die, leaving all my worldly belongings to Sophie. As Dr. Levy draws the session to a close, he instructs me to leave my back pain and my narcissism there.

After the session we talk about what happened. I say: "The visions were so vivid and every detail popped into my mind without hesitation. I was hit in the back in exactly the place where I have had pain for my entire life. As long as I can remember I have

Irrational Medicine

had a chronic lower back pain." Dr. Levy suggests that since I was attacked, which resulted in my death, because I was affluent that today I associate success with dying. Maybe that's why I sabotage myself.

September 18-20, 2003: I am staffing the New Warrior Training Adventure weekend in Ohio. Steven Judith is the leader on this weekend and I have worked with him before. During the weekend, I laugh more and connect with men I haven't seen since the training last year. Several of the men make remarks about how much I have "opened" since last year and how they can really see who I am for the first time.

On Sunday I return home. I take a long hot shower, greet my children, and go outside and sit on the deck with my dog. I am peaceful, focused, and connected to those that mean the most to me. I feel at one with the world and comfortable in my life right now. This happens whenever I do Warrior work.

November 12, 2003: I do another past life regression with Dr. Levy. This time I discover the life of an Indian squaw in 1592. I decided not to marry my love Running Cloud so I could give 100% of my time to my work as the high priestess Running Deer of the Blackfeet. My tribe was decimated by an attack that wiped out almost everybody. I could do nothing to stop it and did very little afterwards. I died feeling like I was useless and wondering why I should even try.

After the session Dr. Levy points out that I am doing "all or nothing" thinking. I am either good or bad. I am either a dramatic all encompassing success or a total failure. When in actuality I don't stop to think that maybe I did what I was supposed to have done. That I brought the teachings and the healing in the way I was supposed to have done it. That I had indeed made a difference but I just wasn't supposed

Irrational Medicine

to stop the disaster. That by doing something toward my goals/purpose everyday I am being a success. I don't have to hit a "home run" all of the time. It's not all or nothing but rather steady progress wins the race.

November 19, 2003: I begin to feel overwhelmed by my emotions: confusion and shock, guilt and shame, depression, agitation and anxiety, flashbacks and dreams.

I see a television ad for a new ADD medicine called Stratera. I go to my family doctor and tell him I want to try the medicine. He gives me a prescription, and I stop at the drug store to get it filled.

November 21, 2003: At my next session with Char she talks me out of starting the new medicine. She says: "You have come too far to stop now. Give it a few more weeks." I agree not to start the medicine, but I am so tired and my motivation to do anything is so low.

Change My Diet

November 28, 2003: Dr. Dominques recommends that I make changes in my diet. She says, "A bad diet deprives the brain of nutrients and can starve the brain by reducing levels of the glucose it uses for fuel. You need nourishment if you are to keep up your fight. Emotional stress, including depressed feelings, can cause or worsen physical disorders, so that you can end up both emotionally distressed and physically ill. For example, your sadness may lead you to pay less attention to your diet, and poor eating can worsen many diseases, including diabetes and a variety of gastrointestinal problems. Poor diet can also lead to increased weakness and fatigue. Feeling depressed leads to self-

Irrational Medicine

neglect. What we ingest in the form of food and drink builds and sustains our biochemical bodies including our biochemical brains. Drink some alcohol. How do you feel? Is your thinking the same as before you drank it? Eat some ice cream. Eat some chocolate. How do you feel? Each of these and many other substances - caffeine, nicotine, etc. – cause chemical reactions in the body and many also cause chemical responses in the brain. As surely as drugs we ingest alter our body chemistry, the food and drink we digest affects us."

Since I have no idea what the right diet looks like I decide to consult with nutrition specialist Dr. Pam Popper from The Wellness Forum. Dr. Popper has me track what I eat for several days before we sit down for our consultation.

December 6, 2003: I meet Dr. Popper at her office where she reviews my food journal for the last five days. She says, "While some foods give us the raw building blocks for repairing and regenerating the aging cells of our bodies, much of the food we eat is used to provide chemical energy that allows us to be active, creative beings. In addition to the chemical energy our cells use as a primary form of fuel, our bodies also use electrical energy. Looking at your chart I see two problems. First you are not eating enough food and second you are not eating the right type of foods. A basic rule of thumb concerning what we eat is: the closer to nature the better. That is, the less the food is processed, the better. Avoid anything that has the ingredients refined sweetener, enriched or fortified, anything with a # after it, partially hydrogenated vegetable oil, MSG artificial sweetener, artificial fats, whey, iodized table salt, caffeine. Also cut out as much as possible sugar, white flour, processed oils, and dairy products. Eat only "real"

Irrational Medicine

living food as nature provides. Your food should be organic, fresh, and unprocessed.

The type and the quantity of vitamins and trace elements we take in through our diets is important with regard to preventing physical illness. A deficiency of vitamins can greatly impair our body's ability to use chemical and electrical energy at a basic tissue level. Any kind of nutritional stress on the body due to protein and calorie malnutrition or to relative deficiencies of essential nutrients can affect the level of vital energy within the physical body. Studies show that the entire range of depressive symptoms improves with omega-3 fatty acids: sadness as well as fatigue, anxiety as well as insomnia, decreased libido as well as negative thoughts. When patients who suffer from depression have more omega-3 fatty acids in their diet, their symptoms tend to be less impairing than those of depressed patients whose diet is deficient. Another common nutritional deficiency is a lack of the B vitamins. Some of the symptoms include: weakness and fatigue, dizziness, forgetfulness, uneasiness, rage, anxiety, depression, mental confusion, impaired intellect, hostility, and craving for sweets. The tendency to cry for no reason is one of the most common complaints. The second is a constant feeling that something dreadful is about to happen. People who are in a "brain fog" are often deficient in B vitamins.

Rather than taking a lot of supplements I like to see people get the vitamins they need directly from the food they eat. So I want you to have a shake for breakfast each morning. It will consist of a special protein powder and will include green tea for antioxidants, brewers yeast to provide the full complement of B vitamins, flax seeds to provide Omega 3 fatty acids, frozen fruit and soy milk.

Irrational Medicine

Furthermore for your body chemistry to work properly you must have sufficient water intake. Dehydration can be a factor to depression. Water also helps to flush toxins from the body through the kidneys."

December 2003: I start drinking the health shake each morning. It is a lot of work to blend all the ingredients together but it doesn't taste too bad. The first day on the shake I have more energy. As I implement Dr. Popper's other recommendations I can feel my vitality start to increase. I drink my daily shake and eat better food with the same zeal that I use to take my antidepressants and Ritalin.

By now the drugs are clearly out of my body but the withdrawal symptoms continue throughout the month of December.

Chapter 12

A Confrontation With GOD

O Lord, give me understanding concerning Thyself, for I cannot understand Thee except by means of Thee.
- Sufi Prayer

January 8, 2004: I start seeing a therapist about a low grade chronic anxiety that I feel. My energy level is the best it has been in years, thanks to my diet, but I feel anxious all the time. My relationship with this therapist is very different. I talk to him more as an equal rather than an all knowing being. I listen to what he has to say, but I don't take everything as the gospel truth. After all, therapists are human beings. Some got lower grades than I did in high school or graduated at the bottom of the programs in which they learned their trade.

February 16, 2004: I see Dr. Dominques and complain about the low grade anxiety that permeates my body. She says, "It has been a while since you have had a large dose of remedy. Lets go ahead and try the large dose again to see what might happen.

February 17, 2004: It is a very tough day. My anxiety level is very high. I leave work early so I can get a Reiki treatment. I am so distraught and anxious Tere can see it in my eyes.

February 18, 2004: My anxiety is so high that I break down and cry at work. It feels as if something is inside of me and wants to come out - like a caged

Irrational Medicine

animal prowling back and forth. I ask God to help me. Then that little voice inside says: "Contact Steven Judith he can help you."

Steven Judith is a New Warrior leader, and I have staffed with him twice in Ohio. He is at ease with ambiguity: he has a comfort with complexity, and he is able to be decisive in the midst of chaos and uncertainty. He treats every man with respect, a decisive professionalism, wit, and an unshakable belief in their ability to heal and be complete. His life purpose is to make a difference in the lives of other men, and he lives it every day.

I send Steven an email about my condition and within an hour he calls me and says he will work with me. It just so happens that there is a Leader Body meeting at his home in Indianapolis this coming Saturday. He says to come at the end of the meeting and those men can stay around and help me out. I call two friends from my I-Group, Mike Leahy and Michael Figg, and ask them to go with me. I have a feeling that this is not gong to be easy, and I need their support.

February 19, 2004: I have a session with Char, and I tell her what I am going to do on Saturday. She is happy for me because she senses that something big is brewing.

February 20, 2004: I have an incredible sense of fear around what might happen on Saturday, but I have seen Steven work and I know that I can not be in safer hands. This whole week has been a series of synchronic events that have drawn me to do this work. The remedy from Dr. Dominques stirs something up inside of me. My Reiki session with Tere doesn't calm me down like it usually does but it leaves me feeling ready to confront something. In my hypnotherapy session with Dr. Levy I discover that I

Irrational Medicine

have some real anger toward myself that needs to be addressed. All of these events push me to have the courage to ask Steven Judith for help. It is also no accident that there is a Leader Body meeting this weekend that will provide a container of top notch men.

I feel as if the Universe has orchestrated all of these events to get me to go through a healing experience. So I am at peace for what I am about to face and know that coming out on the other side will be worth it all.

Steven's House

February 21, 2004: It takes three hours to drive to Steven's house. It is the longest three hours of my life. I have no idea what is bothering me or what is going to happen.

The session starts with a circle of men standing in Steven's living room. After explaining to the group why we have all gathered Steven looks across the circle and asks, "What can we do for you?" I say, "When I was eight years old I was sexually abused by a neighbor, and I am mad about it." Steven, "Who are you mad at?" I say, "My parents for not stopping it, myself for not speaking up, the abuser for doing what he did and God for letting me go through that." Steven, "OK lets look at each one of those. Do you think that your parents knew about the sexual abuse?" After I think for a moment I say, "No. If my dad had known he probably would have killed the guy. He's a police officer. My mom didn't know or she would have told dad, and he would have killed the guy." Steven, "If you parents didn't know, how can you be mad at them?" I say, "You're right, I can't. I am sure they would have done something if they had

Irrational Medicine

known." Steven, "OK, can we take your parents out of this equation?" I say, "Yes." Steven, "Why are you mad at yourself?" I say, "I feel that it must have been my fault. I should have protected myself somehow, I should have been able to prevent it from happening. I should have spoke up." Steven, "But you were only eight years old. Most eight year olds can't speak up to elders. You didn't know what was happening. One of the great traumas of sexual abuse is that the child is made to feel like a partner in the crime. Most child molesters are considerably older than their victims: their lies sound authoritative to children. Abusers often manipulate emotions of the child until the child thinks they are part of the problem. They manipulate the child into secrecy, which forces victims to keep their emotions bottled up. To an eight year old child it can seem unthinkable that such a person could do something so horribly wrong. Can you say it is not your fault?" I have difficulty saying it, but I get it out, "It is not my fault." Steven, "Again." I say a little louder, "It is not my fault. Steven, "Again." This time I yell, "It is not my fault!" Steven, "Can you see how this is not your fault? I say, "Yes, it's not my fault." Steven, "Can we take you off the list of people you are mad at?" I say, "Yes." Steven, "Now, of the two remaining on your list who are you really mad at? I look all around the room, shuffle my feet, and move my body back and forth as I say, "God." I am shocked because I thought for sure the answer would be the asshole who abused me. Steven, "Why God?" I say, "I am angry at him for letting the guy abuse me. He could have stopped it." Steven, "How about if we give you a chance to let God know how you feel? Look around the room and pick someone who can play the role of God." I look around and pick my friend Mike Leahy. They position him on a kitchen chair so he is

Irrational Medicine

looking down on me, from on high, watching everything I do and say but always at a distance. Steven says, "Now I want you to tell God how you feel. Tell him what you are mad about." I can't say a word. I just stand there shuffling my feet back and forth. I look everywhere in the room except at God. Every fiber in my body wants to run out of the house and go home. Steven, "What's wrong." I say, "I can't." Steven, "You can't what?" I say, "I can't tell God that I am mad at him." Steven, "Why not?" I say, "Because I am not allowed to be mad at God. God is perfect. I am not allowed to be mad at God!" Don Jones steps in and says, "Do you think Jesus was the most perfect human being of all time?" I say, "Of course he was." Don says, "Do you realize that Jesus himself got mad at God? Do you know when that was?" After a moment I answer, "Yes, when he was on the cross. When he yelled out: My God, my God why have though forsaken me?" Don, "That's right. Now if it was OK for Jesus, the most perfect person on earth, to be mad at God could it be OK for you to be mad at God?" I think about it for a while, "Yes, it's OK." Don, "All right then turn around and tell God how you feel." I turn around and I look at God and give myself permission to be angry, to let go. "Why did you let this happen to me? How could you let something so terrible happen to a little helpless eight year old boy? What kind of a God are you to let this go on?" The more I talk the louder I get. "Why did you let this happen to me? How could you let this happen, where were you? Where were you when my brother died, when my parent's divorced, when my wife cheated on me?" Screaming as loud as I can, "Where the fuck were you?" I begin to cough and gag so hard that I double over. Then it feels as if someone has hit me in the back of the head with a sledge hammer, and I

Irrational Medicine

drop to my knees. The pain is excruciating and unlike anything I have ever felt before. It feels like the muscles on both sides of my neck are being torn away from my bones. All I can do is kneel on the floor and cry. I stay on the floor for several minutes because the pain is so intense. Once the pain subsides I whisper, "Why should I trust you now?" Why should I trust you now?"

Don helps me to my feet and says, "Just as there are things about its loving mother that a tiny child cannot comprehend: mysteries remain when we try to understand the infinitely superior mind of God. In your pain it is natural for you to lash out at the hideous, unfeeling monster you suppose was God. The God you thought you hated is just a figment of your tormented imagination. It's time you meet the real God – your Healer. Do you want this type of God in your life anymore?" I say, "No, I do not want this God in my life anymore. I want a God who is loving, peaceful, joyful, compassionate and creative. I do not want a vengeful, spiteful God in my life." Don, "Then tell this God to leave." I look at Mike, who is playing God and I say, "Leave me. I no longer want you in my life." He gets down from the chair and leaves the room. Steven says, "Now look around the circle and pick out a man who holds the energy of the God you want in your life." This time it is easy for me to identify such a man. It is Don Jones, partly because of the energy he exudes of compassion, and partly because he reminds me of my grandfather. Don and I stand face to face on the same level and look into each others eyes. I see a man filled with understanding, love, and compassion. Steven says, "I want you to switch places Jeff and you take the place of God, Don will be you. Now looking at him tell him what you want him to know." I place my hand over

Irrational Medicine

his heart and the words that come out of my mouth seem to come from a different source than me, "This is my son, in whom I am well pleased. You went through what you did so that you can help others. I am with you always." Steven, "Now switch positions, and, Don, you repeat back to Jeff what you just heard." Don looks at me and places his hand on my heart. As he looks into my eyes I see God face to face. He says in a gentle but powerful voice, "This is my son, in whom I am well pleased. You went through what you did so that you can help others. I am with you always." As I look into his eyes, I can feel nothing but love. I feel so deeply the love of God and the healing I have longed for. I start to weep, I am free. After a few minutes Steven asks, "Jeff, do you feel complete now?" I say, "Yes, I am complete." Steven, "Did you get what you came for?" I say, "Yes, I got what I came for." Steven ends the process by saying, "I strongly encourage you to think of your healing process as heroic. The work you have done here is amazing. It takes a great deal of courage to face your demons and few men ever take this challenge."

The three hour ride back to Columbus with Mike and Michael seems shorter and much more pleasant. As I recall what happened at Steven's house I am amazed at this work, I am amazed at such powerful men coming together to help each other. I am thankful to God for what I have just gone through.

Feb 22, 2004: Every muscle in my body aches and my joints are painful. My head is stuffed up. I can't get out of bed. My medical doctor calls this a sinus infection. I am so sick that I miss the entire week of work.

Feb 25, 2004: Despite being so sick I keep my meeting with my new therapist. I explain what happened Saturday at Steven's house and tell him

Irrational Medicine

that the anxiety is gone, completely gone. He says, "I always knew that someday there would be an organization that could make us unnecessary." We spend the rest of the hour talking about the ManKind Project and the New Warrior Training Adventure. This is my last therapy session.

Feb 27, 2004: I give up on my medical doctor trying to treat my sinus infection so I go back to Dr. Dominques. I tell her about my experience at Steven's house. She explains: "Your body is reacting to what happened that Saturday. It is cleansing itself of the trauma it has stored. Many people, after experiencing a major loss of some kind, will come down with a cold or flu. This is the body's way of slowing you down and encouraging you to properly mourn the loss rather than continuing with your regular schedule and burying the feelings. If you fail to recognize the connections between the sinus infection and the grieving, and take a cold pill to reduce symptoms and get back to usual activities, then you have lost the opportunity to process the loss, and perhaps more severe physical symptoms may force you to deal with your emotions at a later time." She gives me a remedy to process the experience and relieve some of my suffering.

A Life Reclaimed

March 1, 2004: Something just kind of changes in me. I wake up, and I really do want to live, I am happy. The cloud of depression has lifted off me, and the nightmare is over. I walk around conscious of how not-terrible I feel and that life is actually joyful. I stand up straight, chest out, shoulders back. Over the next few days, I become all right, safe in my own skin. It happens just like that.

Irrational Medicine

As days go by I notice that the extremes in my moods are not as prominent as they have been, and it is clear that a low grade, fitful instability is no longer an integral part of my life. As I enter into the world of more stable moods and peace, I begin to realize that I know very little about it and have no real idea of what it is like to live in such a place. In many ways, I am a stranger to the normal world.

It is hard for me to get used to my contentedness. I am afraid that I might lose this new way of being. I find it difficult to formulate a way of being and thinking in which the starting point is not depression. Depression has for so long been a convenient – and honest – explanation for everything that is wrong with me. Not only am I no longer depressed, I am free from the weight of 23 years of unexpressed grief over the loss of my brother, two bad marriages, and my career setbacks. For the first time in many, many years I am at peace and can live in the now.

I begin to really understand how stagnant my life had been during the time I was taking the antidepressants and Ritalin. The emotional pain of my life had been dulled by the drugs, but the quality of my life had not improved. I can see the steady withdrawal into isolation and indifference that came upon me as I lived with the drugs. It's akin to the deadly sin of sloth. But it wasn't merely laziness: it was a gradual closing down of the world. As I lost interest or pleasure in ordinary activities, my range of activities constricted. I stopped taking chances, I played it safe, and I began to cut myself off from anything that might shake me up – including loved ones. I was in a pharmaceutical coma.

Over the next four weeks I take advantage of my new zest for life. I get my motorcycle fixed. I

Irrational Medicine

haven't ridden it in three years but now I'm ready. I go to the movies three times in a week. I buy the chocolate Labrador puppy I have dreamed about since I was a kid. I stop watching television and spend all my free time with my boys. I am friendly and don't worry about meeting other people. I don't procrastinate or spend money impulsively. I can actually walk into a store and not buy any thing. I love my life.

March 31, 2004: My boss stops by and says we need to talk. When he shuts the door I get a strange feeling that something serious is about to happen. He then proceeds to tell me that in the reorganization my job is being eliminated. This doesn't surprise me at all given my lack of functioning over the past few years. He is using the reorganization as an opportunity to get rid of me because of my performance, a classic move in Corporate America.

As he sits there going on and on about the reorganization trying to make himself feel better about what he is doing, I just tune him out. My little voice starts to tell me that this is a perfect opportunity to write a book, to tell my story, and to help other people break free of depression.

After he reviews my severance package I smile, shake his hand, and thank him. He looks at me like I am crazy. I then proceed to pack up my desk and walk out to my car.

I have never been stronger mentally, emotionally, physically, and spiritually - I have no fear about my future. I now have the sense of controlling my own life. I have a new respect for myself. This is what it must feel like to be let out of prison.

I can't help but be amused by the irony that I am physically reenacting what I spent the last 23

Irrational Medicine

years trying to achieve. First, I reclaimed my physical health by leaving the psychotropic drugs behind and now, today, the Universe is reclaiming my occupational health by "forcing" me to leave behind the world's largest distributor of pharmaceutical drugs. God does have a sense of humor.

Chapter 13

REMOVE THE DEMON AND YOU DO NOT NEED THE EXORCIST

Psychiatrists have tended to lay a smokescreen over the indubitable fact that in the real world it is not hard either to recognize or to treat the large majority of psychiatric illnesses. It would take the intelligent layman a long weekend to learn how to do it.
- The Myth of Neurosis: By Garth Wood, M.D., a British psychiatrist

Today I am totally free of pharmaceuticals: I am more focused, my heart is open, I am in a loving relationship, I am a great father to my boys, and I feel more at peace. Even when my life becomes tumultuous, I am able to find a place of deep inner peace and deep joy. I find life really worth living. Perhaps because, for the first time I have the feeling that I am really living my own life, and it is an exciting adventure. Now I can better understand my suicidal thoughts. It seemed pointless to carry on under the influence of the psychotropic drugs because I was living a life that wasn't mine, that I didn't want, and that I was ready to throw away.

Since getting off the drugs and going through withdrawal, I have spent a lot of time looking at what happened to me. I am amazed at the number of books

Irrational Medicine

written by doctors that are against the use of antidepressants. There seems to be a growing dissent within the medical community about the effectiveness and ethics of using psychotropic drugs.

Looking back at my life, I am amazed I survived. If the drugs were relieving my depression it was only by rendering my brain and mind unable to generate higher psycho-spiritual responses - not by fixing any chemical imbalance. I have come to the conclusion that there were two major factors in reclaiming my life.

The first factor in getting my life back was getting off of the psychotropic drugs so I could have a fully functioning brain. My doctors were so convinced that I had a chemical imbalance that they didn't look for any underlying reasons for my depression. They didn't look for causes: such as coming from a dysfunctional family system, being the child of a divorce, destructive methods of thinking, abandonment, problems dealing with anger, a generally unhealthy psychological environment, sexual abuse, etc., that might have caused the behavior I was exhibiting.

Looking at the medical model of treatment, I found several major factors that combined to keep me in a pharmaceutical coma for 23 years.

Education - Also Known As Marketing

Doctors focus on the biochemical model of depression because that's what they are taught by big drug companies. The vast majority of a doctor's post graduate education comes from pharmaceutical companies' sales reps. Few doctors have more than a basic and superficial training in pharmacology, and most are too harried to keep up with the literature on

Irrational Medicine

effects and side effects of drugs. Drug companies have enormous influence over what doctors are taught about drugs and what they prescribe. Drug companies spend a great deal of money appealing to physicians to win their overall sympathy and loyalty as well as their support for particular products because they must rely upon physicians to get the product to the patient. Many doctors rely too much on information provided by drug companies, which inflate the values and downplay the dangers of their products.

    The drug industry has been the most profitable industry by far year after year. They are subject to the same market pressures for sales as any other giant industry and will take the same extreme measures when their profits are threatened. Toward that goal, drug companies mount sales campaigns to convince doctors and patients to use their products. The drug companies spend millions of dollars every year influencing each doctor, and to convince patients that they have "diseases" that can be treated with the drugs.

    It is an adage within modern economics that advertising actually creates consumer needs. When emotional discomfort or suffering is defined as a disorder it creates business for doctors and drug companies. Psychopharmacology is sold by calling attention to symptoms people might otherwise ignore and creating unwarranted anxiety by labeling such problems as "disease" then offer salvation in the form of a pill. Today pills have replaced psychotherapy as the "hot" and effective treatment. The campaigns to promote "mental illness" have been so successful that, within a matter of a few years, millions of Americans have come to believe that they have "biochemical imbalances," "panic disorder," or "clinical depression,"

Irrational Medicine

and that their children have "ADHD:" all treatable with drugs.

Smoke Screen

Contrary to popular belief, big drug companies spend far less on research and development than on marketing. The pharmaceutical industry has the largest lobby in Washington – with more lobbyists than there are elected representatives in Congress – and contributes heavily to political campaigns.

The industry claims to be innovative, but only a small fraction of its drugs are truly new; most are simply variations on older drugs. For example premenstrual dysphoric disorder (defined as severe premenstrual symptoms) is treated with Sarafem, which is just Prozac in another color at a higher price. Right now psychiatrists are advocating antidepressants for a variety of disorders, from depression and anxiety to eating problems, premenstrual tension, phobias, and obsessions and compulsions. They have become a jack-of-all-trades drug. This in itself should warn us not to trust the claims being made.

The DSM

Psychiatry has become almost completely dependent on one manual, the Diagnostic and Statistical Manual (DSM), a "cookbook" listing symptoms that has replaced science of deductive differential diagnosis. Many psychiatrists use DSM to diagnose patients after only a cursory examination.

Based on the criteria in the DSM, people who are creative, who have a different learning style, or are angry, or sad can easily be diagnosed as having

Irrational Medicine

depression, ADD or Bipolar Disorder. The DSM has a major flaw because it identifies symptoms but makes no attempt to identify the source of a problem. A doctor then treats the symptoms and the true cause is never addressed.

Physiatrists

In psychiatry the dependence on the drug companies is even greater than in medicine in general. The American Psychiatric Association (APA) colludes with drug companies whose interests lie in broadening markets, encouraging long term use, minimizing the dangers of drugs, and belittling alternatives to drugs. The propaganda for this remarkable perspective is financed by drug companies and spread by the media, by organized psychiatry and individual doctors, by consumer lobbies and even by government agencies such as the National Institute of Mental health (NIMH). As a result many educated Americans take for granted that "science" and "research" have shown that emotional upsets or "behavior problems" have biological and genetic causes and require psychiatric drugs. Indeed, they believe they are "informed" about scientific research. Few if any people realize that they are being subjected to one of the most successful public relations campaigns in history. The public needs to be suspicious of the motives of a campaign that encourages them to seek medical treatment and also tries to help doctors recognize depression.
Many doctors bill themselves as experts on the human psyche, but most of them don't know any more about it than you do. And this is every bit as true of the psychiatrist with advanced psychoanalytic training as it is of the non-medically trained therapist.

Irrational Medicine

Being ordinary people, shrinks don't know anything more about finding happiness than anyone else. It's been suggested, in fact, that psychiatrists go into the profession largely to find out what's wrong with their own personalities.

The managed care industry also has had a hand in promoting the use of drugs as a lower-cost alternative to counseling and other forms of treatment for psychiatric problems.

The Drugs Themselves

No psychiatric drug has been shown to be consistently safe and effective for more than a few weeks or months of use. Even after many years on the market, psychiatric drugs are rarely studied to the degree necessary to determine their long-term hazards or usefulness.

As experience has accumulated with the newer anti-depressants (Prozac is the best known one, but there are a number of others) several important facts have emerged:
- In controlled studies they are only slightly more effective than placebos.
- They cause, in a certain percentage of cases, a very disturbing form of agitation called "akathisia" that can produce violent behavior, especially when associated with another of their effects, "disinhibition" or emotional indifference.
- These drugs may also cause psychosis and/or mania severe enough to result in psychiatric hospitalization.
- They are all associated with withdrawal problems that are much more common and severe than has generally been acknowledged.

Irrational Medicine

Pharmaceutical companies are only presenting the bare minimum on their products. Full disclosure is not on their agenda, and who could blame them? They are businesses and their objective is to make and market products for consumers.

For example Glaxo Smithkline Corporation, the maker of Paxil, was ordered to pay $8 million in a wrongful death suite settled August, 24, 2001. Donald Schell, originally from Wyoming, killed himself, his wife, daughter and granddaughter, February 13, 1998, after taking Paxil. The charges in this case were that Glaxo Smithkline had known since 1990 that Paxil can produce suicidal and homicidal reactions in a small number of people and failed to provide adequate warnings to doctors or on their label about this reaction.

Another example, on October 15, 2004 the FDA mandated that all antidepressants must carry a "black box" warning, the government's strongest safety alert, linking antidepressants to increased suicidal thoughts and behavior among children and teens taking them.

The warning reads: Antidepressants increase the risk of suicidal thinking and behavior in children and adolescents with major depressive disorder and other psychiatric disorders.

The agency's action comes at a time when it faces withering criticism for not acting sooner on antidepressants. Congressional investigations have focused on allegations the agency silenced its own employees who tried to raise safety concerns on the antidepressants.

The FDA

Irrational Medicine

People assume that FDA approval and the widespread distribution of a drug - with many patients taking it for months or years - means that long-term studies have found it safe in regard to side effects, drug interactions, dependency, addiction, and withdrawal. However, that is not what happens. Most drug trials last weeks or months – not years – and involve only a few hundred patients. Side effects, even serious ones, aren't likely to be obvious until thousands of people have taken a drug over a number of years. In addition, drug companies fund much of the research used to determine whether new drugs are safe and effective. They fund projects with a high likelihood of producing favorable results. Sometimes, only favorable clinical data are released to FDA investigators. Negative studies may be terminated before they are ready for publication.

The FDA lends authority to the use of psychiatric drugs by approving them. The public is lulled into believing that regulatory agencies are busy at work protecting them. FDA approval does not mean that drug trials have really demonstrated either safety or efficacy. For example, on September 30, 2004, five years after being approved by the FDA, Vioxx, an anti-inflammatory drug manufactured by Merck, & Co. was recalled after a long term reports suggested that patients taking the drug face twice the risk of a heart attack compared to patients who were given a placebo.

Side Effects

Common side effects of antidepressants: autonomic nervous system signs, such as blurred vision, dry mouth, and suppressed function of gut, bladder, and sexual organs, as well as low blood

Irrational Medicine

pressure on standing, weight gain, sleep disturbances, seizures, and impaired cardiac function. They can bring about anxiety, produce or exacerbate psychotic symptoms, and cause delirium. They frequently produce sedation, lethargy and a blunting of emotional responsiveness, although this often goes unacknowledged by psychiatrists.

Since medication-impaired patients often have little or no idea what is happening to them, they cannot point to their drugs as the culprit. Doctors in turn often dismiss their patients "complaints" as irrational or as due to their mental problems rather than to the drugs prescribed by the doctor. Also many drug-induced adverse reactions seem bizarre.

One way to learn about the side effects of psychotropic drugs is to consult the Physician's Desk Reference (PDR). Compiled by drug companies and distributed to physicians, the PDR lists the known side effects of most commonly prescribed drugs. Although most people think of the PDR as a reference manual, it's actually a device to reduce drug companies' legal liability; by issuing a public listing of the known toxic effects of their products, the companies can claim to have informed consumers about these effects, even though few physicians pass the PDR information on to their patients.

Addiction

The antidepressants and Ritalin caused a form of addiction – a form so subtle that neither myself nor any of my doctors could recognize it for what it is. When I would have a good response to the medicine I was leery about coming off medication, out of fear that I would return to my old way of feeling and behaving. When I had a bad response to the medicine

Irrational Medicine

I was told to stay with it or my depression would return. Either way I feared not having the medicine. Addiction is something that you can't stop. I became psychologically dependent on antidepressants because I so firmly believed they were the answer.

Withdrawal

A study in the Journal of Clinical Psychiatry showed that 70 percent of general practitioners and, surprisingly, a third of psychiatrists don't know that significant withdrawal symptoms can occur when people stop taking antidepressants. It is an under-recognized problem because when people stop taking a drug and then develop new symptoms, they can't believe it has anything to do with the medicine because, if they're not taking it, how can it affect them. But withdrawal clearly does happen, though researchers still aren't sure why.

History of Psychiatric Treatment

Psychiatrists have been wrong before when it comes to drugs and their effectiveness for treating "mental illness."

At one time the psychiatric profession claimed that LSD could expedite the psychotherapeutic process and shorten the time necessary for the treatment of various emotional disorders, which made it a potentially valuable tool in the treatment of mental illness. There were studies indicating that LSD-assisted psychotherapy could reach certain categories of psychiatric patients usually considered poor candidates for psychoanalysis or any other type of psychotherapy. Many individual researchers and therapeutic teams reported various degrees of clinical

Irrational Medicine

success with alcoholics, narcotic-drug addicts, sociopaths, criminal psychopaths, and subjects with various character disorders and sexual deviations. LSD was banned by the federal government in 1967.

The street drug Ecstasy was used by physiatrists from 1977 to 1985 in couples counseling under the name Empathy, because it supposedly made it easier for people to relate to each other. Some therapists claimed that a five hour Empathy session was as good as five months of therapy. By 1984 the drug was being used widely among students in the USA under its street name "Ecstasy." The drug was outlawed in 1985.

Biochemical Imbalance

Many professional and lay people today think depression is caused by a biochemical imbalance in the brain even though none of the "imbalance" theories of depression have ever been verified. This dominant biological theory of depression was derived from speculations on how and why medications sometimes seem to alleviate depression. There are no techniques for measuring the actual levels of neurotransmitters in the synapses between the cells. Thus all the talk about biochemical imbalances is pure guesswork. Because most patients initially respond to psychotropic medications, they generally do appear, at least for a while, to be getting better. But like when drinking alcohol or smoking marijuana, it is because the brain is impaired. On antidepressants you feel less emotional suffering because you reach a state of relative anesthesia. A patient is sacrificing a certain level of brain function in return for a blunting of emotional suffering.

So doctors conclude that if a patient responds

Irrational Medicine

to a psychotropic medication, it "proves" the problem is a chemical imbalance or deficiency, probably inherent in nature. But in fact such improvement on medication says nothing about the cause of a person's problems. If aspirin relieves a headache, we do not necessarily conclude that the headache was caused by an "aspirin deficiency."

Suppose someone is playing the piano and you didn't like him doing that. Suppose you force him to take a drug that disables him so severely that he can't play the piano anymore. Would this prove his piano playing was caused by a biological abnormality that was cured by the drug? As senseless as this argument is, it is often made. Most if not all psychiatric drugs are neurotoxic, producing a greater or lesser degree of generalized neurological disability. So they do stop disliked behavior and mentally disable a person enough so he can no longer feel angry or unhappy or depressed. But calling this a cure is absurd. Extrapolating from this that the drug must have cured an underlying biological abnormality that was causing the disliked emotions or behavior is equally absurd.

It's a myth that a great deal of science is involved in the prescription of psychiatric drugs. Medical professionals simply do not understand the overall impact of drugs on the brain. Why would a biochemical imbalance be at the root of feeling very depressed any more than it would be at the root of feeling very happy? And if there were biochemical substrates for extreme sadness and extreme happiness, would that fact make them diseases?

The biochemical imbalances speculation is actually a drug company sponsored marketing campaign to sell drugs. The speculation has also been promoted as truth by biological psychiatrists to

Irrational Medicine

convince patients to come to them rather than to non-medical therapists.

If You're Not Convinced

If you find it unbelievable that the medical industry puts so much credence in mere speculation I challenge you to ask your doctor for solid proof that antidepressants correct a biochemical imbalance. I also invite you to read *Toxic Psychiatry* by Dr. Peter Breggin, or *Let Them Eat Prozac* by David Healy, or *The Truth About the Drug Companies,* by Dr. Marcia Angell, or *Running on Ritalin,* by Dr. Lawrence Diller.

A Word Of Caution

Don't people have a right to escape the anxiety that comes from depression? To use shortcuts if necessary, including sedative drugs? Yes, they surely do. But doctors should not encourage this as a way of life. There are some situations when drugs may truly be necessary. They can be a powerful means of coping until a person can do the serious work of healing. But they are not a cure and these medications are far from perfect. They can take weeks to become effective and are not guaranteed to work for everyone. Sometimes it takes a painful process of trial and error to find an antidepressant that can help. And even when a particular drug does offer relief, it can trigger various side effects – from insomnia to sexual difficulties to a blunting of all emotions. If you choose to use antidepressants do so only for a short amount of time and seek counseling preferably from a psychologist or therapist that don't have a vested interest in your staying on the drugs.

Your first priority should be looking at other

Irrational Medicine

ways to lift your mood and energy such as changing your thinking patterns and your diet. Then begin the hard work of figuring out what your dark emotions may be signaling. In my experience depression is a sign that something needs to change: an unfulfilling job, a dysfunctional relationship, an attachment to past resentments or disappointments. If you take the medication to feel good but don't confront what is really going on, you not only miss the opportunity to transcend the depression, you will be inviting its return.

It's Time

It is a mistake to view depressed feelings as a disease. Depression is an emotional response to life. It is a feeling of unhappiness - a particular kind of unhappiness that involves helpless self blame and guilt, a senses of not deserving happiness and a less of interest in life. A human emotional or psychological state should not be considered a "disease" simply because it becomes extreme. My doctors overlooked or denied the obvious harmful effects of the severe emotional, physical, and spiritual abuse of my childhood. I needed help to recover from a series of oppressive relationships and from the harmful effects of previous therapy, not psychiatric drugs.

Medical doctors rely heavily on pharmaceuticals and are biased in favor of their use. They take the easy route of writing prescriptions rather than the more arduous route of helping their patients find complex long-term solutions to their emotional difficulties. It's time for psychiatrists to return to being physicians – not seers, priests, gurus, or pill pushers, but real physicians. It's time for them to start asking what's really wrong with their

Irrational Medicine

"hyperactive," "depressed," and "anxious" patients, and to start uncovering and treating the causes of their problems – not just hiding their symptoms under layers of dangerous and addictive drugs. It means looking beyond labels such as depression and anxiety, and seeking the causes of despondency, anxiety, and hopelessness. It means determining and treating these causes, rather than masking them with drugs.

Chapter 14

The Key

The greatest discovery of my generation is that a human being can alter his life by altering his attitudes.
- William James

All that we are is the result of what we have thought. The mind is everything. What we think, we become.
- Maharishi Mahesh Yogi

    The second factor in getting my life back was all of the work I did toward emotional healing. I labored under the belief that life would not always be bad, that there was a bottom to my misery. I believed that someday I would have enough body work, Reiki, or hypnosis, read enough self help books or go to enough seminars. I kept trying the next thing and the next thing. I believed that whatever was disturbing me could be found and dealt with. That's how and why I kept going.
    If you keep doing the work to find the real you there is a point where you transcend into something greater. All the medication in the world cannot give you that transformation. The bottom line is "do your work."
    Remember that you are body/mind/spirit, not body and mind and spirit. What your mind doesn't handle, your body will try to resolve, draining spiritual energy in the process. I addressed my

physical needs by changing my diet, drinking more water, exercising, and getting work done that released trapped energy in my body. I addressed my mental needs by attending various seminars and reading self-help books. I addressed my emotional needs by changing the way I thought about life and what I deserved, raising my self esteem and forgiving those who harmed me. I addressed my spiritual needs by seeking a greater connection to the divine.

What Depression Is Really About

Depression is a human response to a wide variety of psychological, spiritual, and even physical factors. It is both a physical process and an emotional process, a disorder of the body, mind, and spirit all at once. Depression is partly in our genes, partly in our childhood experience, partly in our way of thinking, partly in our brains, partly in our ways of handling emotions. It affects our whole being. It displays itself in myriad ways from chronic feelings of sadness to acute feelings of wanting to die. It drives some people to feel suicidal and others to feel murderous. It provides some people an excuse to be needy and demanding in relationships, and it compels others to live even more independent lives.

Some of the physical factors responsible for depression are disorders of sugar metabolism, weakened pancreatic function, nutritional deficiencies, impaired liver, gastrointestinal breakdown, hormonal insufficiencies, and dozens of other purely medical conditions.

Psychological factors can cause depression, such as guilt, blame and anger that is directed toward oneself. Typically, the individual rejects his or her own right to happiness and, especially, to be loved.

Irrational Medicine

The mental component of depression is a particular way of thinking and feeling in response to disappointment and loss. The best solution requires learning to overcome these negative thoughts and feelings. It stands to reason that misguided, self-defeating ideas can only be changed through embracing better ideas.

If you are unable to deal productively with your feelings, either about past experiences or current situations, those unexpressed emotions will find an outlet in either self-destructive behaviors or acting-out toward others. Unexpressed feelings, like termites, are not always apparent, but if you look closely you'll find them just below the surface, bent on destruction.

Some negative emotions are hardwired into us biologically because they enhance our survival. The anxiety and fear we experience following a trauma are nature's way of telling us to take measures to avoid similar traumas in the future. The sense of numbness and the depersonalization that often occur during or shortly after a trauma are most likely the body's way of allowing us to put our emotions on hold until it's safe to sort them out. These reactions may not be fun but they're not pathological.

Feelings of depression that used to be treated as intolerable can be recognized as signals that the individual needs to become aware of the source of stress or disappointment. In this way, depression can function as a motivation and a guide for discovering that something harmful has happened or is taking place. The individual can say in effect, now I know what's making me so miserable. I've fallen into the trap of succumbing to my spouse's anger, or I've again forgotten to take care of my own needs for love, or once again I'm working much too hard. The depressed feelings not only point toward the

Irrational Medicine

problems, they can motivate the individual to find the courage to change his or her life for the better.

The true opposite of depression is not gaiety or absence of pain, but vitality; the freedom to experience spontaneous feelings.

Ways of Overcoming Depression

There are a great number of mystical traditions and spiritual practices, many paths that lead people to wholeness and peace of mind. The ways of finding renewed motivation and inspiration to love life are as varied as life itself. People have learned to overcome depression and to create a principled, loving life through books and contemplation, through romantic love and family life, through nature, through creative work, through exercise, through the healing passage of time, and ultimately through the courage and determination to change their lives for the better. The process can involve an infinite variety of psychological, moral, spiritual, and religious practices. By ethical and moral practices, I mean those that involve respect for the rights of others. By spiritual practices, I mean those that focus on love and the pursuit of higher ideals whether or not they include formal religion or a concept of God.

Your Thoughts

Masaru Emoto, an internationally renowned Japanese scientist, discovered that molecules of water are affected by our thoughts, words and feelings. In his book, *The Hidden Messages in Water*, Dr. Emoto demonstrates the healing power of such emotions as love and gratitude. He discovered that crystals formed in frozen water reveal changes when specific,

Irrational Medicine

concentrated thoughts are directed toward them.

Dr. Emoto mentally projected love to a bottle of water, which was then frozen and later the ice crystals were photographed. The crystals were beautiful, clear and symmetrical. Next, he let the ice in the bottle melt, before directing hate to the water. Again, he froze the water and photographed the ice crystals. The crystals were misshapen, dense and ugly.

Thoughts can cause water to change form. The molecular structure of water is two atoms of hydrogen and one atom of oxygen. The thought influences the atoms making up the molecule, and the response of the atoms creates the form. The purpose of atoms is to express life in form, and the creative vibration of thought directs the form taken by atoms. Since humans and the earth are composed mostly of water, we affect one another with our thoughts and feelings. Dr. Emoto's message is an important one because it demonstrates a practical plan for both personal and planetary growth.

We each experience an inner world made up of beliefs, which have been programmed by our life experiences. And these beliefs generate the thoughts and emotions that manifest all our outer experiences. Self change begins with reprogramming our beliefs, which then generate new thoughts and emotions, which in turn, create new experiences.

Alternative Healing Methods

The politics of medicine are in many ways similar to politics of any sort; power and money are the motivating factors, the forces underlying decisions and governmental law-making. Medical dogma, and its impact on our consciousness, is responsible for the fact that many Americans, until recently, had never

Irrational Medicine

heard of medical options other than those espoused by the dominant medical system. Treatment options such as Ayurvedic medicine, Chinese medicine, naturopathic medicine, homeopathy, medicinal plant therapies, bodywork, and nutrition, if discussed at all, are relegated to the category of "alternative" and dismissed as worthless. Patients who chose to utilize these different modalities are considered daring, foolish, or strange. But holistic approaches can provide solutions. Alternative therapies, when used at the same time as psychotherapy or medication, can sometimes accelerate the results, intensify the process, or otherwise assist in overcoming the problems.

  The track record of Western medicine is outstanding for acute conditions such as pneumonia, appendicitis, or bone fractures it is far from stellar for most chronic conditions, including anxiety and depression. Complementary therapies should not have to be a last resort when all else fails. Instead they should be considered before deciding which treatments to use. Information about alternative treatments for emotional problems is not always easy to find and has never been collected and presented in a form that allows easy comparisons. I was lucky to stumble upon such gifted and helpful healers when I needed them, but most people have no idea that there are any alternatives or adjuncts to psychotherapy and medication and wouldn't know how to make decisions about them if they wanted to.

  Many complementary treatments are based on different assumptions about the causes of psychological problems. For example, mental illnesses might be caused by nutritional deficiencies, environmental sensitivities, allergies, blood sugar problems, fungal overgrowth, functional endocrine

Irrational Medicine

imbalance, biorhythm disturbances, or blocked energy pathways. Treating these causes with natural remedies, physical manipulations, detoxification, and other procedures sometimes provides a more direct, and therefore more effective approach.

There are numerous alternative healing methods, and I certainly didn't try them all. I have reluctantly come to the conclusion that no single key will unlock the mystery of the human condition. For some people it may take one method or a combination of several different modalities. But the goal is to reclaim all of our misplaced parts of who we are and the bottom line is not to stop searching. Your personal healing will operate on its own timetable, difficult to predict and impossible to control.

The treatment approaches and seminars described in this book all capitalized on the mind and the brain's own healing mechanisms for recovering from depression, anxiety, and stress. Approaches, like acupuncture, nutrition, exercise, emotional communication, and cultivating your connection to something larger than yourself, stem from age-old traditions.

Your instincts are important, and should guide you to the therapies that are right for you. Be sure to consider the time frame for results, the type of contact with the healer, what you will be asked to do for yourself between visits, and the costs of treatment. Try to avoid the temptation of seeing any of the treatments as a quick fix for symptoms that probably took years to develop. Real wellness takes time and your participation in the process. Go to a practitioner, a body worker a hypnotist, or whatever modality is available to you. Then live your life and see if somewhere, something has changed. If it has keep doing that modality. If it hasn't, stop and go on to the

Irrational Medicine

next thing. But keep going. You can be free: you can heal, but it's up to you to do it. It's up to you to pursue it.

Take Responsibility For Your Own Healing

There are things that we can do to recover from depression, but it is up to each of us to find the way. Each person is responsible for taking care of their own physical, mental, emotional and spiritual health. If you use medical professionals treat them as hired-help. Question their treatment plan and do not hesitate to fire them if you are not satisfied with what they are doing for you. Always ask yourself: "Am I better off than before I took their advice?" If the answer is no then you have some more questions to ask.

Taking responsibility for your own health is the most important step toward mental health. If you experience depression think like a consumer – not like a patient. Seek out the best opinion/diagnosis you can find, even if that means disagreeing with your insurers, your physicians, or your employer about what level of care is good enough. Think of the work that goes into buying a good car, purchasing furniture or maintaining a yard or home. Isn't your health – particularly your mental health – more important than any of these?

Accept responsibility for your own health and keep your body, and your brain, in good shape, by eating right, exercising, sleeping well, and following common sense health rules. If something goes wrong anyway, spend the time and money necessary to find a good physician who will uncover your problems instead of hiding them with drugs.

Learn as much as you can on your own. When

Irrational Medicine

we take responsibility for our own health and take steps to get in balance, we open the door to new ways of taking in the world around us. This is the gateway to realizing the self without stress, anxiety, or depression.

Many of us are taught (or intuit) that it is not good form to play too active a role in our health care. Questions to doctors should be polite and deferential, acknowledging their superior knowledge and the wisdom of experience. If we are irritated with the doctor's demeanor in any way or left with an uneasy feeling that something is not right we save our gripes for relatives or friends instead of facing the care giver. Such deference to doctors is a dangerous thing.

Physicians who treat patients and their relatives harshly or condescendingly are far more likely to miss a diagnosis than those who listen carefully. I learned the hard way that it's beneficial to the patient to be a skeptic, to listen to the doctors but don't assume that they're always right. Ask them why they prescribe drugs or other treatments. Look up the benefits and risks of treatments yourself, rather than relying solely on your doctor's recommendations. Get second opinions. Become the kind of patient that doctors dread: a fully informed, confident, and assertive participant in your own health care decisions. For too long, American medicine has treated its patients as passive, ignorant, trusting dependents. Break that habit, insist on being a full partner in your own care, be assertive; remember that it's your health at stake, not the doctor's.

FINAL THOUGHTS

Throughout this experience I have learned how marvelously the mind can heal, given half a chance,

Irrational Medicine

and how patience and gentleness can put back together the pieces of a shattered world. But before I could completely heal, before I could love unconditionally, I first had to stop the war within myself.

Life can be so overwhelming, yet there is hope. Take responsibility for yourself. Work on raising your level of consciousness, because if you want to get something more out of life than what you are now getting, you must become a different person. Life only gives back to you a reflection of your level of consciousness. It's like this. If you wish to see the view from the first level of a building, you cannot see it from the ground level: you must go up to the first level. When you are tired of the view on the first level and want to go and see what is on the second level, you must again raise yourself up to the second level. Consciousness is also like this. You will only see what is on your level of consciousness.

I am not a fortune teller: however, I can tell you one thing about your future, and that is, if you don't change yourself today, you will get tomorrow more or less the same as what life served you yesterday. The future for most people is usually a reflection of what they got in the past, albeit in another form. To change the future, you must change yourself in the present moment. It is in the present moment that all change occurs.

You will achieve freedom from depression momentarily, lose it, and then go after it again. Eventually it sinks in. It's worth it: keep trying. It's critical for you to hold an absolute intention for yourself to heal, regardless of what goes on around you, or what others might offer you in the way of discouragement or "getting real."

The key question through all of this is **"Are you**

Irrational Medicine

relying on the drugs to fix you?" If you are then your primary focus needs to be giving up the idea that the answer lies in a pill. You need to get up and find a way to get to the bottom of the issues and get your life back. Like it or not, if we want to get better we have to change ourselves, and to suggest that it can be done simply and easily is insulting. Recovery from depression is hard work. You must demand to live in a better world.

Irrational Medicine

"Do you know nothing is more important than that you be joyful and joy-filled? Joy is your reason for choosing to come into this lifetime. It is literally your reason for being, in your current physical body. You did not choose, at your soul level, to come into this lifetime to experience anything except joy. There is obviously much in your world today that, if you focused on too much, would not bring joy. But it has always been thus, as long as you, as a human race, have walked your beloved Planet. You have always been free to choose what you want to focus on. Which, therefore, means you're free to EXPERIENCE whatever you focus on. No one -- not even a whole world -- has any power to create your experience for you. You -- and you alone -- create your experience, your own reality. Your choice to focus on the positives -- and there are many more of those than there are of the negatives -- will ensure your joy. That choice will also ensure your remaining fully connected to your Higher, wiser Self. All is well, my dear ones."
- Chief Joseph, of the Nez Perce tribe